THE ARTS IN MEDICAL EDUCATION
A PRACTICAL GUIDE
SECOND EDITION

T0210409

ELAINE POWLEY
*Medical Educator, Yorkshire and
the Humber Postgraduate Deanery
and University of Leeds, UK*

ROGER HIGSON
*Medical Educator, Yorkshire and
the Humber Postgraduate Deanery
and University of Leeds, UK*

WITH

DAVID POWLEY
*Freelance Theatre Practitioner,
Group Trainer and Drama Therapist*

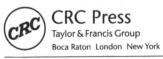

CRC Press
Taylor & Francis Group
Boca Raton London New York

CRC Press is an imprint of the
Taylor & Francis Group, an **informa** business

Radcliffe Publishing Ltd
33–41 Dallington Street
London
EC1V 0BB
United Kingdom

www.radcliffehealth.com

© 2013 Elaine Powley and Roger Higson

First edition 2005

Elaine Powley and Roger Higson have asserted their right under the Copyright, Designs and Patents Act 1988 to be identified as the authors of this work.

All rights reserved. No part of this publication may be reproduced, stored in a retrieval system or transmitted, in any form or by any means, electronic, mechanical, photocopying, recording or otherwise, without the prior permission of the copyright owner.

British Library Cataloguing in Publication Data

A catalogue record for this book is available from the British Library.

ISBN-13: 978 184619 565 5

The paper used for the text pages of this book is FSC® certified. FSC (The Forest Stewardship Council®) is an international network to promote responsible management of the world's forests.

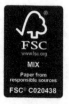

Typeset by Phoenix Photosetting, Chatham, UK

CONTENTS

PREFACE TO THE SECOND EDITION

This book is intended as a practical guide for those wanting to find out how an enhanced experience and appreciation of the nature of the arts can be applied to medical practice. It is about using the arts as a resource in medical education, and it is written as a handbook that can be conveniently referred to and used as a manual in teaching.

It is not an academic text that has reviewed all of the literature about medicine and the humanities, nor is it a book about art appreciation or literary criticism.

The authors, Elaine Powley and Roger Higson, are experienced medical educators, and David Powley is a drama practitioner. The content of the book is based on our experience in using the arts in the postgraduate education of general practice registrars (trainees) and in working with their trainers.

We started using the arts in teaching because we saw them as a way of getting to the heart of those transactions in human discourse that make up good practice, by enabling an imaginative understanding of another person's feelings and recognising the diversity of human behaviour and its consequences. We saw the arts as a way of retaining the balance in everyday medical practice between, on the one hand, applying scientific knowledge and procedures and, on the other, engaging with the patients' own stories, beliefs, demeanour and experience of illness, and the influence of their culture and environment.

We wanted to share our passion and enthusiasm for the way in which the arts awaken sensibilities and open pathways to intuition and perception – the way in which creativity enables you to cross boundaries, connect, synthesise and celebrate curiosity and enquiry about human activity, all of which can inform action.

We discovered that practitioners attending our courses often departed happy, excited and fulfilled. They said that they had been able to start thinking widely, and had found the feeling parts of themselves that had been submerged under the accumulated silt and debris of mechanistic thinking. Old concrete was breaking up, and flowers growing through the holes.

In Part I we talk about the *principles and methods* of using the arts in teaching. We introduce each area of the arts, and then in individual chapters we discuss the *attributes* of the different art forms – literature, poetry, music, paintings, photography, drama and film – and show how to use each form in teaching, giving examples of practical exercises and tasks, and how to facilitate responses. We discuss the *application* of these gained insights, perceptions and knowledge to medical work, and their *relevance* to patient care.

In Part II we build on these principles and methods and explore how the arts can be used in what are sometimes viewed as difficult areas of the medical curriculum. Finally, we take three arts resources to reinforce the concept of the breadth and depth of material which can be found and used creatively in medical teaching.

We hope to signpost your travels.

Elaine Powley
Roger Higson
January 2013

ABOUT THE AUTHORS

Elaine Powley was a general practitioner in Kirkbymoorside, North Yorkshire for many years and has worked in medical education as a GP trainer and programme director. She has taught widely on postgraduate seminars for the Academic Unit for Primary Care, University of Leeds. She is a member of the European General Practice Research Network and has presented papers relating to using the arts in medicine. She is a passionate traveller.

Roger Higson qualified in medicine at Cambridge University in 1971 and was a general practitioner in Masham and Kirkby Malzeard in North Yorkshire for 30 years. He is currently a training programme director on the Northallerton Training Scheme for General Practice and runs seminars on using the creative arts in medical education in the Yorkshire and Humber Deanery and the Academic Unit for Primary Care at The University of Leeds.

David Powley was, until 1991, Head of Drama, Film and Television at York St John College in York, where he helped to set up an honours degree programme and where he also co-founded and was director of a postgraduate dramatherapy training course. He has been a practising state registered dramatherapist since 1980. He has worked extensively in educational contexts, in the community and in organisations as a trainer in drama (both text-based and improvised) and therapy. Since 1991, he has worked in these fields internationally as a freelance.

We would like to acknowledge the contribution of those doctors who have attended our teaching sessions, and thank them for their generosity of spirit, creative energy and enthusiasm in embracing a different way of learning.

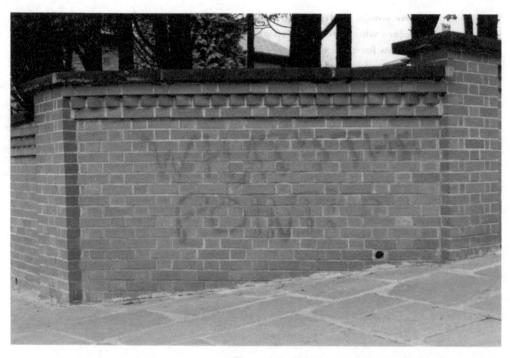

Figure A Graffiti, University of Leeds Campus, Artist unknown

WHY USE THE ARTS IN MEDICAL EDUCATION?

George Taylor

WHY SHOULD WE HAVE MEDICAL EDUCATION BASED ON THE ARTS?

A more sensible question is probably 'Why not?'. We live in a real world full of emotions and unexpected happenings. Doctors, whether they like it or not, are sometimes viewed by the general public as 'super beings', people who can cope with all their problems without it affecting them. We all know that this is not true, that we all have human frailties, that every day at work at least one situation arises that tests our ability to cope. Sometimes in these days of protocols and evidence we could be forgiven for thinking that primary care's greatest challenge, dealing with uncertainty, has been overcome. Just apply the evidence, develop the protocol and – hey presto – the patient's problem will be solved! But we know that some areas of primary care are evidence light, that people are all different, that their presentations do not always fit the protocol, and that they can cope or not cope with ill health to different degrees. We also know that these characteristics apply to doctors just as much as to patients. Because of this, it becomes clear that anything that helps practitioners to perform better and to understand and cope with their daily working world has to be of major advantage. This is where using and enjoying the arts in education can really come into play.

Recognising the role of the arts in medical education, particularly in primary care education, is not a new phenomenon. *The Future General Practitioner*, one of the most important publications for general practice in the 1970s, identified the special knowledge and skills required to practise successfully in primary care. It also clearly identified that, because primary care is about people not diseases, primary care education should base itself firmly in the arts. Since that time, major changes have taken place medical education at all levels in the UK. Although undergraduate medical education has in the past been likened to five years of being spoon-fed lots of facts, interspersed with short periods of regurgitation of these facts to help assess progress, major changes have taken place. These developments in the undergraduate medical course have seen massive progress towards a more realistic educational experience. Many schools have moved to problem-based learning, and some have even recognised that medicine, traditionally entered by achieving high marks in science subjects, has a great deal of 'the arts' involved in it. There are now many examples in medical education of educational modules based around the place of the arts in medicine.

Postgraduate training has perhaps surprisingly lagged behind undergraduate education in using the arts in education. Half-day release programmes have recognised the different way in which problems have to be viewed. A patient-centred approach that recognises the place of social and psychological as well as physical factors associated with disease has clearly become the norm. Perhaps this is why it is sometimes disparaged by hospital doctors and trainees for going into the 'touchy-feely' world rather than providing 'proper' scientifically based education about diseases. However, what has been lacking in postgraduate half-day release programmes is the regular use of the arts as an educational methodology, although some educators have recognised the value of the arts and use them regularly in their teaching. Salinsky in London has a high input of arts-based teaching and, for example, gets his trainees to read and discuss novels in relation to a variety of clinical situations. He provides a good example of an educator who has clearly recognised that the arts par excellence can be used as a tool, a pathway, through which to develop greater understanding of individuals, to understand their reasoning and reactions, and better to understand ourselves. At the end of the day it's all about how people tick.

This book is an example of the benefits enthusiasts can bring to an organisation. It is based on the work of two Yorkshire educators, Elaine Powley and Roger Higson. Recognising the value of their personal use of the arts in the education they were providing for their own GP registrars and registrars on their local training schemes, they came together to run a regular seminar for GP educators in Yorkshire. This is recognised by those who attend as providing valuable development for themselves, both in their knowledge and skills about the arts and also in how to use them as educational tools. There is always the concern that they may only be attracting like-minded educators to their courses, which although popular and well attended may be attracting a very skewed audience. I do not believe that this is the case, but perhaps we should call their seminar 'Diabetes mellitus, the scientific basis, some complex cases' one year and see how it goes with a surprised 'scientific' audience?

More recently, the authors have extended their sphere of influence, having developed a very successful module for the Leeds University Masters degree in primary care, a qualification aimed at a multi-professional primary care audience.

As with all good ideas, the reasons for their success become obvious when you just stand back and look. What is primary care? It is not about diseases, but about people. People are not machines, but are thinking emotional beings. However, they are complex beings, and for the individual to unravel his or her own emotions for him- or herself is sometimes difficult. For health professionals trying to understand them, skill is frequently required even to work through their complexity to get to the real person and their problems. Often the practitioner also needs methods to cope with these problems when they have been identified.

We know that adults learn best when the subject is seen as real and relevant to their everyday needs and they can then see rapid value for their everyday work. The arts are such a broad canvas for learning that using only a few of them can be as beneficial as attempting to use a huge range. For example, I personally cannot comprehend what people see in most opera or much modern art, but that does not matter as I still have access to so many sources of learning in the other arts. Popular music, which is often thought of as simplistic and superficial, has provided me with educational insights based on its lyrics. Specific songs have also been of great value at times of personal stress. I have learnt a great deal from the wonderful insights into human nature in the books and plays of Alan Bennett, in the writing of Monica Ali about the Bangladeshi community, and in the work of Roddy Doyle about working-class Irish people, particularly the gentle history of his parents' life. In my former role as a GP in a mining community in north-east England, a variety of books (both fiction and non-fiction) have helped me by developing my understanding of the lifestyles of the British working class. At a different level, John King's *The Football Factory* gives a terrifying insight into how some young working-class males live.

The examples are endless, and although in my own case they can be found predominantly in literature, music and film, for someone else it might be in soap opera, pop music and magazines, and for others, in opera, classical music and poetry. The use of any or all of these reveals that the arts can be used to stimulate thinking, to provide emotional support and to help to identify parallels and insights into everyday life. They can help any involved professional cope with, for example, the effects of giving bad news, including the effects on themselves, on the involved patient, and on his or her friends and families The arts have a role at times when professionals are feeling low because they have failed to achieve their own personal high standards. In the longer term, they may help to avoid 'burnout' in the primary care workforce.

So enjoy this book. I hope that it will stimulate you to discover or develop the ways in which you can use the arts in education. I am sure that if you do, your teaching and learning will move into a new and more fulfilling dimension.

George Taylor
Formerly Director of Postgraduate GP Education,
Yorkshire Deanery

REFERENCE

Royal College of General Practitioners (1972) *The Future General Practitioner: learning and teaching.* RCGP, London.

PART I

Part 1

1 SETTING THE SCENE

Read the two extracts which follow. The first is from a medical textbook, and the second is from the recreated true story *The Perfect Storm* by Sebastian Junger. Both describe drowning.

'Drowning is death by suffocation from submersion in any liquid. Wet drowning involves significant aspiration of fluid into the lungs. This causes pulmonary vasoconstriction and hypertension with ventilation/perfusion mismatch, aggravated by surfactant destruction and washout, reduction in lung compliance and atelectasis. Acute respiratory failure is common. The onset of symptoms occurs rapidly. Dry drowning, a small amount of water entering the larynx causes persistent laryngospasm, which results in asphyxia ,and an immediate outpouring of thick mucus, froth and foam, but without significant aspiration.'

Oxford Handbook of Accident and Emergency Medicine

'The instinct not to breathe underwater is so strong that it overcomes the agony of running out of air. No matter how desperate the drowning person is, he doesn't inhale until he's on the point of losing consciousness. At that point there's so much carbon dioxide in the blood, and so little oxygen, that chemical sensors in the brain, trigger an involuntary breath whether he's underwater or not. It's called the "break point". It's a sort of neurological optimism, as if the body were saying "holding our breath is killing us and breathing in might not kill us, so we might as well breathe in". Until the breakpoint, a drowning person is said to be undergoing voluntary apnea, choosing not to breathe. Lack of oxygen to the brain causes a sensation of darkness closing in from all sides, as a camera aperture stopping down. The panic of a drowning person is mixed with an odd incredulity that this is actually happening. The process is filled with desperation and awkwardness. "So this is drowning." A drowning person might think "so this is how my life finally ends".'

The Perfect Storm

For safe medical practice it is essential to know the scientific information contained in the first extract. What happens in the novelist's account is that the physiology of drowning becomes an identifiable human experience. It is a person who drowns – you can feel how it must be, you can relate with it. You could be there.

The novelist as artist has created a bridge between science, on the one hand, and humanity, on the other. This can start the process of gaining intuition by understanding the experience of illness, and not just the biological condition accompanying it. There is the opportunity to realise the emotional effect of medical events.

In this book we shall look at different art forms to open up safe crossings. We shall provide the opportunity to stand on the bridge, to see what it feels like and continue to the other side.

You will find images and text throughout the book, which do not have explanations or instructions. This is deliberate and will allow you to reflect and be creative in your own interpretations.

- To obtain an overview of the book read the next section **'Territories of the imagination'**, which will signpost your travels.
- To find out *how* to teach using arts resources, read the chapter, **'Teaching with the arts'**.
- To find out in detail about using **individual art forms** and the exercises you can try, read the subsequent chapters, each of which deals with a specific art.
- Practical exercises in each chapter appear in blue.

Although the learners referred to in this book are doctors undergoing postgraduate training in primary care in the UK, and their trainers, what we describe in the text is transferable to medical education in any healthcare discipline and any culture.

TERRITORIES OF THE IMAGINATION

LITERATURE AND NARRATIVE

"'I ran into a snake this afternoon," Miss Shepherd said. "It was coming up Parkway. It was a long grey snake – a boa constrictor possibly. It looked poisonous. It was keeping close to the wall and seemed to know its way. I've a feeling it may have been heading for the van." I was relieved that on this occasion she didn't demand that I ring the police, as she regularly did if anything out of the ordinary occurred. Perhaps this was too out of the ordinary (though it turned out that the pet shop in Parkway had been broken into the previous night, so she might have seen a snake). She brought her mug over and I made her a drink, which she took back to the van. "I thought I'd better tell you," she said, "just to be on the safe side. I've had some close shaves with snakes."'

So starts Alan Bennett's *The Lady in the Van*. This is the story of himself, the community he lives in, and the woman who chose to live in an old van, eventually parked on his driveway. The book describes the daily events of her life and the impact on those around her. In doing so it debates the nature of tolerance, dependence, eccentricity and humanity, and questions the boundaries that define mental illness. It is an easily read short account, with chronological entries much like those in a medical record. However, this is far more that a factual case history in its ability to record all the aspects of Miss Shepherd's care and management.

During a tutorial, a doctor training in General Practice reflected, after he had read this book, about an old lady he had been visiting regularly and whose demeanour of poor response had puzzled him. He now understood what might be going on in her world, and as a result how he could better communicate with her. His agenda for her care was suddenly much wider.

Go to: Chapter 3   It's my story

Punctuation
Question mark
Full stop
Semi-colon
New paragraph.

This poem was written by a doctor just before her appointment with a surgeon to discuss treatment of her recently diagnosed rectal cancer.

Poetry is not the usual language of the consultation. However, it is a way of distilling the essence of a feeling, an idea or an experience into a satisfying shape or wholeness that, like a good painting, encompasses everything about a moment, often with the use of metaphor. Patients use metaphor all the time – to set the scene, and as a way of trying to describe what they are experiencing ('My headache is like a hammer pounding in my brain').

People also turn to poetry in times of need or intense emotion. You don't necessarily go to poetry for answers, but the process of reading or writing poetry can help to you think and to feel your way through difficulties and anxieties. Memorise a poem, and it can be summoned up again if the need arises.

Go to: Chapter 4   The language of feelings

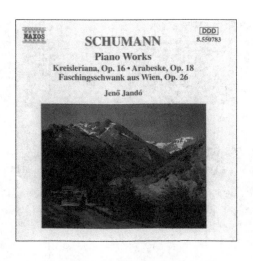

Figure 1.1 Schumann Piano Works

Music appears to be an essential ingredient to most people's lives. Why? We do not know, except that it is pleasurable, and it can soothe, relax or excite. Music has been written at times of distress, emotion and celebration. It can accompany events, so making them more significant and more memorable. Music often expresses feelings and releases emotions in situations where words are inadequate.

Peter Maxwell Davies wrote a haunting melody, *Farewell to Stromness*, when it appeared that the nature of his Scottish community would change if plans for mineral extraction went ahead. This piece says more than words can express.

Opera is a sung story, in which music is the vehicle for carrying the dialogue and expressing an outpouring of human experience and feeling, in dramatic and exciting circumstances. The arias and the tunes, are memorised, and whenever heard again, are familiar reinforcements of a particular feeling as well as in themselves profoundly satisfying.

A scene in an opera, because of the effect created by the music and the voice, can rapidly portray vast scenarios of the depth of human suffering, elation, love.

Go to: **Chapter 5   Sound sense**

Figure 1.2 *Steep Lane Baptist Chapel, Yorkshire* (1976) by Martin Parr

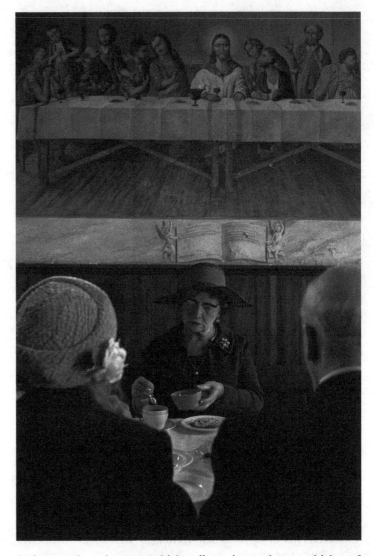

Artists produce images, which tell stories and are vehicles of identity, representation and truth. Art is a kind of shorthand which endeavours to portray everything about a scene, or people, in one single image. Artists have the need to express what is inside them and what has been stimulated by their reaction to their outside world, be it shapes, beauty, human activity, or to create in an abstract way an explanation of some feeling.

Go to: Chapter 6   A way of seeing

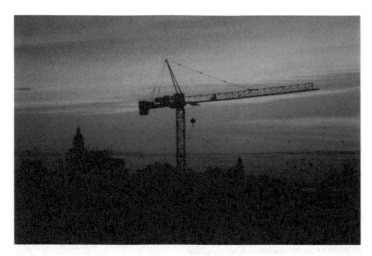

Figure 1.3 Sunset over Brussels

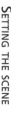

13

The appreciation of form and function, the nature of beauty, and the reasons why aesthetics are important and significant are not normally included in a medical curriculum with a scientific basis. Yet we daily observe the changing aspects of the human body and we are attuned to the significance of a different outline or a new shape. This is seen in our environment. Examples are all around us. To respond to it you need to be there and acknowledge its impact.

Go to: Chapter 7 Out on location

FILM

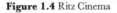

Figure 1.4 Ritz Cinema

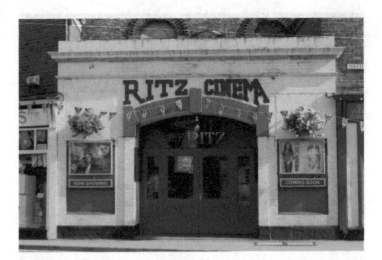

Picture a wild beach in nineteenth-century New Zealand, with crashing surf. Alone on the beach a woman and child are crouched by their possessions in wooden crates, including a piano. Coming through the bush to meet them are a landowner and his Maori workers. This man and woman are to marry. They have not met, and the woman has been unable to speak since she was 6 years old, although she can hear. 'Silence affects everyone in the end, but I don't feel silent because of my piano.' Her new husband will not permit the piano to be carried from the beach with them. He does not have enough porters, he does not perceive its importance to her, and he assumes that she would rather have the crates containing her clothes. As they leave the bay, all that is shown on the screen is the piano, alone on the sand, surrounded by the empty landscape, and with the noise of the surf and wind.

This is a scene from the film *The Piano*, directed by Jane Campion. It portrays a story which debates conflicts, passions and boundaries. When watching a well-made film, we can be transported into its action and become part of the story as we react with the characters, also feeling distress, anger or joy at what is happening, or wanting them to do it differently because we perceive alternative solutions.

There is an opportunity both to learn about our own responses and at the same time to analyse how people communicate or miss cues, and what their subsequent actions or dilemmas, expectations or beliefs are.

A woman doctor in a group discussing the above film extract said: 'That was me, when I arrived at Heathrow from India, with my bags and only knowing how to use a stethoscope.'

Go to: **Chapter 8   Take one**

DRAMA

... And everyone can do it.

Do what?

- Tell stories about ourselves, because for all of us every day is a series of little narratives, so there is plenty to tell.
- Turn the stories into playlets, sharing in the process the pleasures of working creatively with others and the experience of mutual support.
- Discover how much more we can learn about ourselves and others by being physically involved in the action, in expressing relationship and feeling.
- Explore what each story can tell us of who and how we are, and how useful such knowledge of ourselves and others can be to us as professionals.
- See how working with scenes from existing play texts can expand our understanding of our own and our patients' experience.
- Learn how the actual process of working through drama can strengthen qualities and attitudes of mind useful to the way in which we conduct our professional lives.

Go to: Chapter 9   The drama of everyday life

2 TEACHING WITH THE ARTS

In this chapter we start you off on a journey into new educational territory. We outline the principles involved in teaching with the arts. We describe feedback, some of the challenges we have encountered, and how participants are assessed.

'Those that do teach young babes
Do it with gentle means and
easy tasks.'
Shakespeare, *Othello* Act II,
scene 2

Any teaching session that uses the creative arts needs a structure which contains practical exercises based on arts resources, to enable learners to participate, to develop ideas and try them out. The structure must also accommodate forums for consolidating and summarising insights and perceptions gained, and allow discussion about their relevance in the day-to-day medical world.

A teaching session is like a play in acts (*exercises*). Introduce the theme (*your aim*) and characters, the set and the story (*the resource*), allow people to get involved with it and have moments of high drama and quiet reflection (*engagement*), work towards an ending which produces explanations and resolutions (*facilitation*), and provide opportunities for a sequel (*application*).

HOW TO DEVELOP THE STRUCTURE OF A SESSION USING AN ARTS RESOURCE

'The course had a skeletal structure, on which I was able to hang my experiences.'

1 HAVE A CLEAR AIM

There should be not only an overall educational aim for the teaching session, but also a clear idea why an arts resource will be the most effective way of achieving it.

2 FIND AND SELECT A RESOURCE

What can arts resources offer?

In selecting your resource, whether it is a painting to look at, a piece of literature to read or an extract of a film to show, you need to think about what responses it might engender, and what their relevance is for personal and professional development in the topic that you are planning to explore. Think about those things that artists explore and exemplify, and which can be discovered by using their work. For example:

- diversity in human behaviour and personality
- human relationships
- emotions and feelings
- life events
- culture and environment
- communication.

Throughout the book we give examples of resources we have used. However, we do not include a comprehensive list of novels, paintings, music, poems and films that you can use. This is deliberate. We believe that it is part of the development of the creative process for the teacher to select and pick their own. It is good to have read the book, heard the music, found the poem or been to the exhibition. This probably means developing a regular habit of seizing opportunities for visiting arts venues, and being alert to and aware of possibilities.

You can choose material that you read, view or hear critically, with an *aim in mind*, once your senses are alerted to this process. You can reflect on your own responses and how to awaken similar insights and enthusiasms in learners.

However, we can suggest *pathways* to resources, and remember there is a lot of the arts about!

1 Read reviews in the arts sections of newspapers. Follow up anything that sounds as if the theme would be relevant.
2 Look at Internet websites for museums and galleries – find out what's there. Go and see for yourself.
3 Read the monthly *Sight and Sound* magazine (published in the UK), which gives a synopsis and review of every film released for public viewing, and video and DVD releases. Plan your cinema visits.
4 Browse in bookshops, and go to other sections as well as fiction.
5 Watch out for documentary programmes about the arts in the media; plays and opera that are being broadcast. Extend your portfolio by trying something that you initially thought might not be up your street.

3 DESIGN AN EXERCISE USING THE CHOSEN ARTS RESOURCE

This involves being creative and imaginative. The guiding principle is that the exercise must enable the learners to work out and experience for themselves those ideas and feelings you are trying to elicit. In subsequent chapters you will find exercises which we have designed and used in teaching sessions. These can be used as a starting point. You will find that the exercises themselves spark further creativity, and the process develops a momentum of its own.

4 ACHIEVE ENGAGEMENT

The *setting* must be conducive to this type of learning. You need a space which is correctly ventilated, free of clutter and quiet, and which can be appropriately adapted to the planned activity (this is discussed in more detail in Chapter 9, 'The drama of everyday life').

Present your material in a stimulating, exciting and, above all, creative way. The resource is giving you a way in – without it you cannot get hold of the feelings and ideas you are hoping to explore.

Engagement occurs if the resource is appropriate, interesting and presented with enthusiasm and passion. This enables learners to begin to cross the bridge into the world of creativity, to start thinking in an open and imaginative way, and to release ideas which foster *more* creativity.

Be aware of the gradual awakening and enlightenment that need to come before action in some learners, in contrast to the immediate response of others, who want to give it a go at once.

5 FACILITATE RESPONSES

This is about picking up cues from your learners' responses, interpreting and developing the ideas that are produced.

> 'It was refreshing and personally enriching to have the human side of ourselves allowed expression in a supportive environment.'

It may be necessary to direct learners' observation or listening, by specific but open prompting such as the following.

- 'What is this about?' – this is a non-threatening way of questioning their understanding.
- 'What does this do for you?' – this begins the exploration of feelings and emotions.
- 'What does this remind you of?' – this promotes discussion of the learners' own experience and new intuitions.

The facilitator should be aware that significant feelings and emotions may be released during this work. These should be acknowledged, their meaning clarified and action taken to make them understandable, so that when a similar emotion is engendered in another situation, the learner is more able to cope, having benefited from *this* experience of dealing with it.

Sometimes the group may produce ideas in response to the resource which you had not anticipated, which are totally different from your own ideas, and which indeed you had not even thought of. You can only work with what you are given – find a way of using these ideas, and do not give in to the temptation to follow only your own curriculum and thus miss potentially interesting issues. Curiosity helps. You might say: 'That's new to me, you're taking me down a path I had not seen. Tell me more.'

Teaching is a dialogue, and in hearing creative responses, which after all is the process you are hoping for, you get something to work on, and in return your own ideas will be looked at with interest.

What comes out of a session may lead on to further ideas – more creativity!

6 APPLICATION TO PROFESSIONAL AND PERSONAL DEVELOPMENT

This is about landing after flying high and visiting a new and very different country, reclaiming the baggage of everyday life, unpacking the souvenirs of the journey and thinking about how they can be used effectively.

> *'I can see how this fits in with my work – it will help me understand what patients are trying to tell me and what I should say next.'*

FEEDBACK

> *'It was a very challenging experience. I spent a lot of time out of my comfort zone, finding myself having to perform in front of peers, writing lines of poetry (initially quite frightening, ultimately satisfying). In many ways I became aware of my own limited abilities with regard to the necessary vocabulary to describe what I was seeing and feeling. At times I struggled to find relevance to my everyday practice and teaching, until the final session. Here the exercise of actually sitting down and planning some teaching while thinking about incorporating the arts and everything we had done, brought it all together very well – yes it can be done, yes it is desirable, yes I want to give it a try.'*

There are two areas you are interested in.

1 Comments about the teaching session/course itself – addressing its content, the resources used, the quality of the presentation, the style of the teacher and group work, and the setting.

2 Reflection about the personal experience of the learner, and how it was for them – their overall feelings, opportunities for active participation, discovering learning needs, any changed perspectives, their own development, insights gained and relevance to their work are all important for you to hear about.

So ask learners to:

- recall details of their experience
- reflect upon their feelings
- record what they think they have learnt.

The process of thinking through and writing a feedback/evaluation piece in a narrative way enables learners to consolidate and summarise for themselves what it was all about, and to give meaning to the experience. On a longer course this might take the form of a reflective diary.

'I have realised how a knowledge and appreciation of the arts helps us to touch our own humanity, and can be applied to develop empathy with patients.'

'I have been able to go to places in myself that I would not perhaps wish to visit alone.'

'I am amazed at my creativity and that of others. We start our careers so full of ability and potential and then get crushed by the pressures. I will certainly change the pattern of my teaching, restructure my holidays and weekends, and I'll write more poetry (I used to).'

In obtaining feedback you can find out if your aims were met, what worked well and why, whether any areas need changing and whether any new ideas need to be introduced. Your own teaching style and presentation skills may need to be refined.

There will be some learners who stay within their known boundaries of factual and familiar thought (sometimes known as 'concrete thinkers').

Feedback can sometimes be negative. You need to be prepared for this and be able to respond to it. Some aspects can be challenging, especially if such feedback arises in the middle of a group session.

'I can't see why watching a feature film has anything to do with medicine. I mean it's just someone's idea, and it might not have been like that at all. It's a waste of time.'

There is a challenge to engagement here, and the facilitator has to find some way of not getting stuck, recognising their own sense of exasperation at this apparent blinkered, 'only-in-the-tracks' thinking, and the confrontational, aggressive nature of the learner's statement. And not, as the messenger, get shot!

The learner's feedback may be a defensive reaction to an unknown world, an attitude which the facilitator must penetrate sensitively, providing some intermediate safe areas for the journey. The learner's response may indicate a failure of imagination, a lack of curiosity, a lack of desire to see an alternative view, or preoccupation with the facts that they are accustomed to using. These are attitudes, which may benefit from being changed.

You could respond to this as follows: 'Thank you for bringing this question up. You are obviously finding some difficulty in finding relevance of this exercise to your work. It is an interesting point to consider. Can I ask you to consider something you had to do for the first time that was unfamiliar? How did you set about it?'

Members of the group may offer suggestions that give insight into their different learning styles. This will illustrate that things can be done in different ways, but with the same aim. Would a different approach have been more successful? Is someone else's method worth considering? How do we learn from experience?

This approach may help the 'dissenter' to start thinking laterally and to see the facilitator as a guide who can take them on some different routes, albeit with a map. The facilitator will also have appreciated more about that person's learning needs.

ASSESSMENT

There may be occasions when you are required to make a formal assessment of your learners. You are assessing:

- evidence of personal development
- ability to observe
- changes in attitude and approach
- development of flexibility
- ability to respond, interpret and apply with empathy.

This can be done from an analysis of:

- reflective diaries
- creative work produced
- level of participation during teaching sessions.

It is the taking part that is important, and what it can lead people on to, both in themselves and as professionals.

What's good about teaching with the arts?

- The enjoyment of working in a creative way.
- Being imaginative and using many different approaches to teaching.
- Using resources which are interesting, compelling and beautiful in their own right.
- Experiencing the enthusiasm, excitement and joy of learners as they become involved in creative work and benefit from it.

The following poem was written by a doctor following a seminar on the use of the creative arts in medical education:

From the ribs of the upturned hull
seasoned by many crossings
the wounded healer
sees, as if for the first time,
green garlands of weed and
bright splinters of shell;
senses, as if for the first time
cool currents, and soft breeze
in the heat of the day
hears the great waves
in the heat of the day and the
moonlight
and knows his frail craft,
moored under the moonlight stars
worthy of travelling wider oceans.

Sheena McMain, 2000

3 IT'S MY STORY

INTRODUCTION

'All happy families are alike but an unhappy family is unhappy after its own fashion.' This is the opening sentence of *Anna Karenina* by Leo Tolstoy, one of the greatest stories ever told. It is the story of humanity as it unfolds within a family, and it explores many life events, including love, passion, marriage, adultery, abandonment, parental anxiety, psychosomatic illness, death by suicide and the search for the meaning of life.

All of us have a story to tell – usually not as dramatic as a great Russian novel, but all the significant events in our lives start with 'Once upon a time'. Even this book is part of the story of its authors' lives.

Our lives are constructed along a storyline which is partly pure autobiographic non-fiction but partly a fictional and edited version of real events. These stories are narratives and help us to make sense of what is happening to us both physically and mentally. The telling about events gives meaning to the experience.

In this chapter we shall look at the nature of narratives and their value as a resource in teaching. Understanding narrative is an especially important aspect of teaching communication and consultation skills. The ability to communicate is enhanced by hearing the narrative of a medical encounter, and diminished by being concerned only with information and fact gathering. We shall look at how narrative gives meaning to experience, and engages the imagination to release perceptive and creative responses. In the end we wish our learners to achieve narrative competency by allowing the patient's tale of apparently disconnected events to unfold, and then being able to interpret and respond in a way that is related to the patient's own experience.

'We live our lives forwards but understand them backwards.'
Søren Kierkegaard,
Danish philosopher
(1813–55)

NARRATIVES

Medical narratives are the stories doctors and patients tell.

Patients' narratives, written by patients themselves, are stories about illness from the patient's perspective, including the effect it has on their life, their feelings about the illness itself, and their feelings about doctors and about treatment. These narratives also attempt to give meaning to illness, to explore the reasons for the unfolding, seemingly unexplained and puzzling events. Narratives have a beginning. They are set within the context of patients' lives, they interpret biophysical models, they are concerned with implications and consequences, they are layered with feelings and emotions, and they extend over time.

Doctor's narratives are stories written by doctors about patients under their care. They may illuminate and give insight into the patient's predicament and suffering, but most importantly they illustrate the doctor's own feelings. In this way they are more than the notes written in a patient's case record or chart, which may only contain factual information about the patient's disease.

Fictional literature is a rich source of patient/doctor narratives. Later in this chapter we shall use the novels *Regeneration* by Pat Barker and *The Woman Who Walked into Doors* by Roddy Doyle to describe the use of literature-based narrative in medical teaching. Fiction is a window on to the world – a mirror of human behaviour and experience – and it may give penetrating insight into human feelings and emotions. It provides the opportunity to venture into the imagined lives of others. It exposes the reader to situations which might only be encountered after very many years in practice, or which might not have been recognised. By its very nature it stimulates the imagination and encourages the reader to think beyond the obvious.

Narrative also occurs in other art forms – it is not the exclusive preserve of the written word. You will see this illustrated in the chapters on image ('A way of seeing') and music ('Sound sense').

Narratives contrast with **clinical histories**, which are the day-to-day records written by health professionals in a patient's case notes or charts. Increasingly formalised and mechanistic, they are boxes to be ticked on forms or templates to be completed on computers. They are a bare catalogue of facts – words and numbers recording symptoms, signs, investigation results, diagnoses and treatment plans, words which are increasingly turned into numbers, scores and rankings. Clinical histories are written often without a pronoun, making them even more impersonal. Referral letters have become pro formas. Clinical histories are doctor-centred and tend to create a logical story or sequence of events. An extreme example of the clinical history is the death certificate, where there are no clues as to what lay behind the diagnoses, or what contributory factors there might have been to that person's illness, such as violence, bereavement, poverty or inadequate healthcare. They tell us nothing about the person who has died.

Clinical histories, being a story or record of the attention given to a particular illness or pathophysiological sequence of events, are thus in sharp contrast to the illness narratives described above, which are concerned with those things that cannot be measured or counted, and give an account of the sufferer's subjective experience and locate the significance of the illness within their life history. Clinical histories tell us about the patient but not about the person.

USING NARRATIVES IN TEACHING

Using the creative arts in medicine, whether for education or professional development, is all about understanding human behaviour, the human predicament in sickness and in health, and thereby facilitating medical encounters. The study of narratives can be used as part of this process and helps us to:

- understand the patient's experience and make sense of illness by constructing stories
- understand the listener's response to stories
- gain deeper insight into the patient's experience
- connect better with patients and thereby develop empathy
- facilitate reflective practice
- enhance listening and interpretive skills
- give meaning to the patient's experience
- enhance and promote writing skills
- understand the value of therapeutic writing.

How can we use narrative material, whether it is written by patients or doctors or found in literature? There are no prescriptive right or wrong methods. Most of the teaching scenarios described below have developed creatively during seminars and teaching sessions. Ideas spawn ideas. Teaching sessions using the creative arts should be self-regenerating.

PRINCIPLES OF TEACHING USING WRITTEN NARRATIVES

The process is as follows:

> Read → discuss → Facilitate and analyse
> responses → discuss applications

Reading

Allow enough time for the group/individual to do the pre-course reading and suggest the learners think about the following questions.

• What is the story about.?
• What effect has it had on them as a reader?
• How does it relate to medical practice?

Discussion

Emphasise that the exercise is *not* literary criticism. The book/story is not being rated good or bad. However, some insight into the structure of stories and different styles of writing will inevitably emerge during the discussion.

Facilitation

The aim is to engage the whole group, to encourage reflection, to pick up cues and expand on responses, and to promote discussion and debate. Use open prompts such as: 'How was this for you?'.

Record on a flip chart the salient points which arise from the discussion. These can be amplified, and they provide useful summary cues at the end of the teaching session. The main focus should be on the meaning of the narrative both to the reader and to the characters within the story. It is very much a 'What is happening at this point?' approach.

Application

It is important to locate the teaching session in reality and to encourage the group or individuals to see its relevance to their everyday work, whether clinical practice, teaching or personal development.

PRACTICAL EXAMPLES OF NARRATIVE RESOURCES THAT YOU CAN USE

Here are some narratives that we have worked with and to which we have applied the principles outlined above.

LIFE AFTER A MASTECTOMY BY VERONIQUE MISTIAEN

This is a narrative written by a patient about her experiences following mastectomy for breast cancer.

'Sitting in my bath, I show my reconstructed breasts to my children. "They are massive," says Alec, eight, fascinated by all the scars. "People won't look that closely. They won't know," says Zoe sweetly. She is 11, her own breasts just a hint. After a pause, she asks in a little voice, "Am I going to have breast cancer, too?".

I lost my breasts to cancer last winter at the age of 42. The previous summer, on Independence Day, I learnt that the lump I had felt in my left breast for two years, the lump my GP had repeatedly told me nothing to worry about, was an invasive breast cancer. The minute I found out, I felt different. The energetic working mother I thought I was dissolved into a terrified patient in a world I knew nothing of.

I had a lumpectomy and several lymph nodes removed from my armpit, followed by six months of chemotherapy, which left me bald and weak. Then I learnt the cancer was more aggressive than first thought, so I would need more tissue removed. I also found out that I had a higher risk of developing cancer in the other breast. After a painful discussion with my husband, I decided to have a double mastectomy with immediate reconstruction.

My surgeon at the Royal Marsden Hospital (on the NHS) did a beautiful job. "It's a miracle," my mother, who had a mastectomy without reconstruction years ago, exclaimed when she saw me after surgery. But it's not the same. My breasts look great – I can wear all the clothes I used to, even a bikini – but they don't feel like my breasts. They are harder and unyielding, and I keep wondering what people must think when they hug me. Alec, who likes to snuggle in my arms when reading, complains they are "not cushy enough".

I feel ambivalent about my breasts. They have lost most of their erotic power – they brought me cancer, were looked at by doctors, discussed and cut and I have little feeling in them. Yet, I still feel like myself, sometimes sexy, and I love them for the life-affirmation they represent. Jean-Paul, my husband, keeps reassuring me, "you look beautiful. You are still the same – all I care about is for you to be all right. Nothing else matters …". And he tries to show he means it. My friends, too.

Life is strange. I remember reading about women having a mastectomy and thinking I could never bear that. But as with many things, when you are confronted with it, you have no choice, you somehow adjust and move on. The mastectomy itself hasn't affected my self-image that much – I could almost convince myself I had cosmetic surgery – but the reason behind it, cancer, has. I sometimes felt tainted because I had cancer. I cannot trust my body the way I used to, and the tamoxifen I have to take for the next five years reminds me that the future is still uncertain. I never used to be preoccupied with my looks, but now I often scrutinize my face in the mirror, looking for changes – worried.

I am now healthy and working again. I walk outside and feel the wind in my hair. It is an incredible feeling. Not even a year ago I was wearing a hat and spent days prostrate on the sofa, unable to do anything, even read. I sometimes feel so happy that I can skip and sing on the street.

Our life is normal again and we enjoy it more. We cherish what we have, brush aside the inevitable irritations and are perhaps more tolerant. But deep down, in each of us, there remains a sediment of fear and sadness. It creeps back in different ways. Jean-Paul and I still wake up every night around 4am – the anxiety hour. Zoe and Alec seem to quarrel more and request a lot of attention, almost as if they needed to make up for the time I was not there for them.

"Mum, I wish you didn't have to have cancer," Alec told me a few weeks ago. "Oh, me too," I answered. "But it's gone, I am fine now."

"Yes," he said, "but you cannot do what you used to do – I remember you used to collect me from school and swing me in your arms, you used to roll about with me in your arms. Now you can't because of your bad arm" (the surgery left my left arm numb and weaker).

"It's true, but it's not such a big thing," I answered, a bit surprised. "I know, but I miss it," he whispered, his eyes full of tears.'

This story illustrates some of the salient features of a patient narrative – it is not just a record of medical events, it describes her feelings and the effect of the experience on her whole life. Topics which might arise from a story such as this are:

- the medical aspects, e.g. reaction to missed diagnosis by her GP, initial severity of the cancer underestimated (opening to question the reliability of medical expert advice), more aggressive surgery required, personal decision-making by patient and husband.
- the uncertainty of living with cancer
- flags of illness (constant reminder due to the need to take medication every day)
- body and self-image

- sexuality
- the effects of illness on family; declared or covert fears of children whose parents are ill
- the patient's feelings when confronted by a potentially fatal disease
- irrevocable life events
- the use of metaphor in illness narratives
- content – has she concentrated on these aspects of her illness?

The task of the facilitator is to enlarge upon these topics and to help the group to understand their relevance and application in their day-to-day professional lives:

'Let us explore the question of self-image. How has the patient expressed her feelings about this?' She is initially very objective and complementary about her breast reconstruction, but then talks about her ambivalence about her breasts with an undertone of anger and sadness.

'What should this tell us about our management of patients who are facing mutilating surgery?' The discussion could be broadened into considering patients undergoing facial surgery, patients having stomas or even patients who have sustained severe burns.

'How does she express her uncertainty?' 'The energetic working mother I thought I was dissolved into a terrified patient in a world I knew nothing of … the Tamoxifen I have to take for the next five years reminds me that the future is still uncertain … but deep down, in each of us, remains a sediment of fear and sadness.'

'Let us look at content. How do we explain that different aspects of the same illness are important to different patients? How can we recognise this? How is this important in our care of patients?' Narratives are the unique stories of individuals, who try to weave perplexing events and feelings into the tapestry which is the rest of their life. If we do not recognise what is important for a given patient, if we do not follow their storyline, then we will end up in a therapeutic cul-de-sac.

THE BLIZZARD BY MIKHAIL BULGAKOV

This narrative was written by newly qualified, 25-year-old Mikhail Bulgakov, who was sent to practise medicine in the depths of rural Russia. This was 1916 when there was no running water and no electricity, and in the winter horse-drawn sleigh was the only form of transport. The story is about a visit, requested by another inexperienced doctor, to a young woman dying following a head injury. There is a blizzard, and wolves are about. The patient dies shortly after he arrives.

> **Get your learners to read this story.**

This narrative might be used to help young, inexperienced doctors when they are faced with clinical responsibilities shortly after they have finished their training. What similarities are there between the challenges faced by Dr Bulgakov and those in their own professional life? Might it be a way in for them to voice many of their feelings and anxieties about life and work as inexperienced medical professionals? This might include, for example:

- inexperience and responsibility
- delegation
- appropriate qualification and training
- lack of resources
- fear
- feelings of inadequacy, especially when confronted with inevitable death
- duty
- the fact that doctors have feelings
- the importance of reflection, especially after a traumatic (significant) event.

The story might also be a vehicle for discussions about more immediately clinical matters, such as out-of-hours and emergency care in remote areas and in adverse weather conditions, the appropriate management of the patient who, on first encounter, is obviously on the point of death.

Bulgakov covers a wide range of topics which, despite advances in medical science and technology, are still very relevant to present-day practice. Doctors are still human beings, with feelings and emotions, innate and unlearned but still to be understood. The study of narratives can bring students and young doctors closer to these human aspects of medicine.

THE WOMAN WHO WALKED INTO DOORS BY RODDY DOYLE

This fictional narrative is about abuse within a family. Set in the gritty world of modern Dublin, it challenges us with raw language, images of domestic brutality and medical blindness. It tells the life story of Paula Spencer, a battered woman. We learn about her childhood, adolescence, infatuation with Carlo – at once violent and loving – and her marriage, with its many beatings and visits to casualty departments where no one asks the question she craves:

> 'The doctor never looked at me. He studied parts of me but he never looked into my eyes. He never looked at me when he spoke. He never saw me. Drink, he said to himself. I could see his nose twitching, taking in the smell, deciding. None of the doctors looked at me ... I didn't exist ... They stared at the bruises for a split second, then away, off my shoulder and away ... The woman who wasn't there. The woman who was fine. The woman who walked into doors.'

This is a patient's unfolding story, fragmented and moving backwards and forwards in time as in real life. It is disturbing and unsettling. It can be used to explore the theme of domestic violence, doctors' attitudes to this problem, its effect on children, its manifestations and its concealment, When used in this way, learners want to discuss the following themes:

* the use of crude language
* adolescent behaviour (especially sexual)
* family dynamics
* domestic violence
* doctors and abused patients
* women and alcohol
* doctors' behaviour, especially towards frequent attenders
  who may be drunk.

These topics, which are so vividly described in the book, fire the imagination and get learners engaged with real-life problems. They provide insight not only into the patient's perspective of what is happening to them, but also their perception of stereotyped medical behaviour – the disinterested doctor.

> 'Ask me.
>   I'd have told them everything. I swear to God I would have. If they'd asked. I'd have whispered it. If they'd asked first. He pulled my arm behind my back and lifted me off the floor. It would have been easy after that, watching them listening. He hit

me. He kicked me there. He burned me here. He did it. He did it. Save me. I'd have told them everything. I just had to be brought behind the curtain, asked the right question.'

There are also passages in the book which are free-standing narratives and powerful resources for teaching. For example, the opening of the book with its description of a young policeman trying to tell Paula that her husband, Carlo, had been killed, is a brilliant portrayal of inexperience and awkwardness, and could be used to help doctors seeking advice about breaking bad news.

REGENERATION BY PAT BARKER

> Ask your learners to read *Regeneration* as pre-course work, and come prepared to talk about the main themes that run through this fictional narrative.

The story is set in Craiglockhart Hospital, a treatment centre for the victims of shell shock during World War One. It contains vivid descriptions of the effects of shell shock and the dialogues of Dr WHR Rivers with these patients, including the poet Siegfried Sassoon. Fiction blends with characters and events, which have a historical basis.

The facilitator should have a very clear picture of the book and its themes. It is a good idea to have made notes on each chapter and to include the main topics that are likely to be discussed. You may decide to look at the book from particular standpoints – for example, the doctor (Rivers), the patient or general themes:

Doctor themes
- Dilemmas of diagnosis and treatment, especially when there is a political agenda. Does this have resonance with today's health service?
- The convenience of a diagnostic label. Sassoon could avoid being court-martialled by having a psychological explanation (diagnosis) for his actions.
- Relationships with patients. The difference between the ones you like/have something in common with and those with whom you have a personality clash.
- Exhaustion/burn out, and knowing when to rest. The perils of self-diagnosis.
- Conscientiousness and duty.
- Working with colleagues.

- The burden of shouldering patients' problems.
- How the doctor is perceived by the patient.
- Evidence of humane responses beyond the immediate need for them.
- Inhumane treatments and issues of consent.
- The case report – what the doctor chooses to disclose.
- Difficult consultations (especially with the character Prior).
- A doctor as a patient (the character Anderson).
- Being faced with information (Sassoon's poetry) which the doctor has not had to process before.

Patient themes
- The need to be evasive. Lying in order to avoid facing up to issues.
- Hostility and aggression.
- Guilt about the doctor's reaction.
- Wanting to be loved – parent/child relationship with doctor.
- Emotional repression.
- Relationship with the doctor and its boundaries.

General themes
- The importance of feelings in medical encounters.
- Homosexuality and its 'treatment' in the early twentieth century.
- Poetry – refuge or active therapy.
- The use of metaphor (e.g. medicine as a battlefield).
- Relationships – the similarity between officers/men and senior/junior doctors.
- Post-traumatic stress.

What happened in an actual teaching session
A group extracted these themes from the book as powerful topics for discussion.

1 The book was disjointed, with several different stories running through it. Is this intentional? This parallels the experience of doctors listening to a seemingly incoherent patient narrative during a consultation.

2 The conflicts between duty and action as a doctor – in this case making people better so that they could return to the front line and be killed.

3 The personal cost of being a doctor – Rivers becomes ill as his patients recover.

4 'Baggage' – many of the characters in the book carry considerable baggage, which is manifested in the opaqueness

of some of the passages when things are not straightforward and clear emotionally.

5 Loneliness – of the patients in their misery and guilt, despite close contact with comrades in the hospital.

6 Professional isolation of Rivers – he is geographically along way from his roots (i.e. Cambridge and London), and seems to have little in common with his colleagues at Craiglockhart in Edinburgh.

7 The different relationships Rivers has with patients of different classes – he befriends and colludes with Sassoon and takes him to his club, but he is outwardly hostile to Prior. Doctors *do* use different language and exhibit different behaviours with different patients.

8 The 'male mother' concept, rejected by Rivers, but a powerful image necessitated by men being thrown together in difficult circumstances and having to look after each other.

9 Relationship between officers and men – a possible parallel to that between senior and junior doctors.

10 Homosexuality – never openly discussed, but hinted at obliquely. Could this be used as contemporary metaphor for our public and private personas?

11 Relationship between Sassoon and Owen, who is not really developed as a character in the book. Does he act as a vehicle for Sassoon's development? This is a universal aspect of human behaviour.

12 Poetry – Rivers learns after initial incomprehension that this is a distillation of emotion and has been used therapeutically by Sassoon.

The group, which consisted of medical educators, then discussed these themes and suggested the following ways in which *Regeneration* could be used in teaching:

- The book could be viewed as a series of narratives and consultations and be used to promote consultation analysis (*see* the exercise below).
- It raises the problem of the health and well-being of doctors, especially when they are burdened by emotionally traumatised patients. How can this be addressed?
- The modification of doctors' behaviour in response to different patients.
- It is also a very effective text on which to base teaching about post-traumatic stress disorder. The accounts are graphic and

not easily forgotten, and they engage the imagination in a far more dramatic way than a bland textbook description of the condition.

Using the narrative in *Regeneration* to teach about consultation

Ask your learners to read the description of Rivers' second encounter with Prior (in chapter 6) and describe what is happening in this meeting, and to consider whether there are any parallels with consultations that they may have had with patients. You might wish to emphasise the following points.

- The description of Prior's *body language* (arms folded over his chest and his head turned slightly away).
- Rivers' *questioning*, which is direct, blunt and displays antipathy (refer back to their first meeting in chapter 5, which was full of conflict).
- the *effect of Prior's voice* on Rivers' attitude to him (forming impressions about patients), some *shared understanding* (both would prefer to be elsewhere).
- Rivers' reaction to being questioned and challenged by Prior.
- Rivers picking up clues (*'Are you in despair?'*).
- Rivers' reaction to Prior's refusal to talk (i.e. to engage in the treatment that he recommended), his retraction and *negotiation* about hypnosis, and the *effect of an interruption*.

The nature of narrative can be further explored by doing exercises in creative writing, using clinical histories as a starting point. These encourage participants to think beyond the clinical facts, to engage their imagination and to try to transport themselves into a patient's mind and to view situations and problems from that perspective. This essentially reflective exercise may give a new insight into a previously unconsidered view of a patients illness/ disease; and may also offer insights into the doctor's own way of thinking and behaving.

PRACTICAL EXERCISES YOU CAN TRY

A VISIT TO THE HAIRDRESSER

This is a useful introductory exercise which emphasises the difference between *fact* and *story*, and how, by concentrating on information-gathering alone, the whole essence of a situation may be missed. It is used to illustrate the power of narrative.

> Ask each member of the group to remember their last visit to the hairdresser and recall a list of factual information about the event (e.g. where, when, cost, type of cut, name of hairdresser, next appointment). Share this information as a group.

Then divide the group into pairs, who will tell the story of their visit to each other, including what really happened during that visit to the hairdresser, the true circumstances of the visit, why the visit was made on that particular day, at that time, to that particular hairdresser, what was talked about, what was the salon like, who else was there and what was the hairdresser like. What was the experience really like?

This has enabled the participants to discover in a non-threatening and non-clinical setting the nature of storytelling – the narrative that lies below the surface of any encounter.

The task of the facilitator is to bring out aspects of human behaviour and to challenge assumptions made around seemingly straightforward sets of data.

These ideas are developed in two further exercises, which involve learners creating narratives from patient records (which can be real or fictitious). These encourage an imaginative approach to storytelling, to give meaning to and deeper insight into the experience of illness.

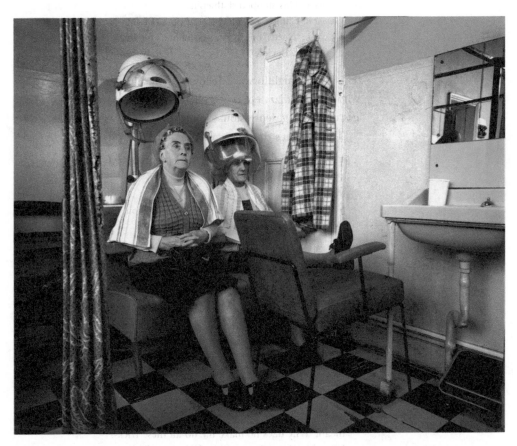

Figure 3.1 *Spending Time* (1986), by Martin Parr

THE PATIENT RECORD

Participants are asked to bring a printout of the computer record of a recent consultation with a patient and to write a creative patient narrative – the story which lies behind this consultation.

For example:

Complaint: Dizziness present.

History: Having 2–3 attacks/day lasting couple of seconds to 5 minutes. Varying times. No warning. Has fallen a couple of times. Feels OK afterwards. Work involves heights. Doesn't drive. Has stopped dothiepin.

Comment: Clinically could be petit mal. Advised at risk so shouldn't work. Needs hospital assessment, so refer. MED 3 issued to patient. Review 1/12.

This is a straightforward follow-up consultation about a woman who has had dizzy episodes. There is a background of possible but not convincing depression.

The patient's **doctor** wrote the following **patient** narrative:

They're still coming – attacks out of the blue. Will I fall wont I?
What's happening?
Why me?
Work don't seem interested in me as a person.
Why me?
Does anyone care?
I've written this list of when and where as I was asked but what does it mean. Perhaps it means I will lose my job?
He keeps asking me for details but there is no more. A pattern? No. Loss of control? Maybe. What do I think it could be? I don't know. He's the doctor.
I know I'm falling but compared with my accident this is nothing – not even bruises.
What will happen to me?
Does he think its all in my head? How can it be?
Why don't work understand? After all it's just dizziness. Who does it hurt? Not me! But why is it happening? What do these questions mean? Why does he make me do all these tricks?
Why doesn't he do something? He just talks!
I'm not scared – but why are they happening? Why do I need the hospital?
But he knows best.

The doctor was surprised at what he had written and how he had written it.

The exercise had given him the opportunity to reflect on

aspects of the case that he had not realised were significant for the patient. He gained insight into the patient's predicament which he had not previously possessed, including:

- her need for more explanation and clarification
- the implications for her of her symptoms – both now and in the future
- her concern about her work and apparently unsympathetic employers.

Why was the story written in a staccato questioning style? Maybe this was a reflection of the doctor's uncertainty. Perhaps it reflected the pressure of the patient's need to know.

The exercise highlighted all the things the patient wanted to tell the doctor but was perhaps unable to. The underlying insecurity and vulnerability of this still wounded patient are understood. The difficulty that the patient experienced in expressing her feelings in words is emphasised by the powerful use of metaphor.

THE HOSPITAL LETTER

This is a fictitious letter from a physician to a colleague. We have written it in a deliberately factual mode. The content could be altered for any given clinical scenario.

Dear Doctor

Re: Mr Leopold Bloom

This 57 year old man was admitted as an emergency under my care recently following a 'funny turn', for which we have found no cardiac, neurological or metabolic cause. He had been drinking heavily and is under some stress at home.

He has no significant past medical history. He has been taking citalopram for some time. He has a family history of diabetes and ischaemic heart disease.

He smokes 40 cigarettes a day, takes little exercise and is overweight. His cholesterol was 8.2 and BP 180/110. We noted a possible Parkinsonian tremor.

He seemed reluctant to consider lifestyle modification. He has been started on medication according to the enclosed schedule, with an appointment to be seen in the neurological clinic about his tremor in due course. I have not arranged further general medical follow-up.

With kind regards.

Yours sincerely

Dr Thomas Gradgrind FRCP
Consultant Physician and Pituitary Endocrinologist

> The participants are asked to write the 'true' story of this
> episode in Mr Bloom's life from:
>
> 1   the patient's perspective *or*
> 2   his wife's perspective *or*
> 3   his daughter's perspective
>
> An X-ray or pathology report could be used as an alternative
> starting point for this exercise.

THE WAITING ROOM

A final exercise in narrative asks learners the question 'What is
the patient's experience when consulting a doctor?' It asks them
to consider what is it like to be the person in that situation,
what are they thinking about, what their concerns are, and **what
it feels like to be the patient**. This exercise demands that
learners use their imagination and helps them to explore some of
these questions.

> Learners (trainee practitioners) are asked to sit anonymously
> in a doctor's waiting room, to observe patient behaviour and
> then to choose a particular patient around whom to construct
> a first-person narrative, which gives the patient's thoughts and
> feelings while waiting to see the doctor.

This exercise encourages the trainee practitioner to glimpse the
inner world of a patient. It also provides the trainer with some
insight into the learner's own thinking and personality.

One learner recently wrote:

> 'It's really busy in here this morning. Why does everyone look at
> me when I come in through the door? … An obvious father and
> son combination across the way are called. The boy is limping, the
> lady next to me laughs and queries a football injury. I don't think
> he is the type for football … Why do people seem so surprised
> that it is busy first thing on a Monday morning? I can almost
> see them assessing themselves as to whether they feel unwell
> enough to stay or not. No-one leaves! … In bundles a mum with a
> pushchair and two children – I just know they will sit next to me
> as the toy box is dangerously close: they do! I should have shuffled
> along when I had the chance … This boy is manic – if he keeps
> bumping into my legs I will have to say something. She seems
> oblivious to it, more concerned with singing incey-wincey spider
> to an uninterested child, and how can she have confidence to sing
> in front of a room full of people?'

The piece displays interpretive skills and imagination – the ability to paint a word picture from images. This is a self-conscious, uncertain patient, who is uncomfortable with close contact with children. Is it a self-portrait with pointers to be picked up as training progresses? (This might also be a powerful tool teach about the organisation of waiting areas and the importance of the environment in which medical encounters take place (*see* Chapter 7, 'Out on location').

CONCLUSION

The exercises and workshops described in this chapter have been designed not only to encourage and develop practitioners' interpretive skills, but also to promote imagination and creative thought to get inside what the patient is experiencing and suffering – to enter their world and engage with their emotions. This will in turn foster empathy, intuition and understanding of both self and the patient.

In the next chapter we move the storytelling process a stage further and look at poetry as a means of interpretation and communication when the language of prose seems inadequate.

REFERENCES

Barker P (1992) *Regeneration*. Penguin Books, London.

Bulgakov M (1995) The Blizzard. In: *A Country Doctor's Notebook*. The Harvill Press, London.

Doyle R (1998) *The Woman Who Walked into Doors*. Vintage, London.

Mistiaen V (2002) Life after a mastectomy. *The Times*. 6 February.

Tolstoy L (1954) *Anna Karenina*. Penguin Books, London.

4 THE LANGUAGE OF FEELINGS

POETRY AND METAPHOR

The last chapter was all about stories – the stories of people's lives and how these are interpreted and recorded. In this chapter we shall develop the narrative theme and explore poetry as a means of expression where conventional prose seems inadequate. We shall discuss how this is often achieved with metaphor and words that require a leap of imagination and intuition, and how poetry can be used as a resource in teaching about difficult areas in medicine and can in itself be therapeutic.

No particular expertise is required to appreciate the ability of poetry to communicate something very powerful, but, for many, poems are an unfamiliar and alien territory. Recall how, in chapter 2 of *Regeneration*, Rivers the scientist reacted to the poems Siegfried Sassoon had given him when they first met at Craiglockhart Hospital.

> 'Rivers knew so little about poetry that he was almost embarrassed at the thought of having to comment on these. But then he reminded himself they'd been given to him as a therapist and not as a literary critic.'

You can respond emotionally to a poem without knowing how this effect has been technically achieved.

Rivers is not alone in his anxiety. Poetry is often considered to be difficult and inaccessible, but there does seem to be a natural resonance with this art form, as evidenced by radio and television programmes in the UK about poetry (*The Nation's Favourite Poems, Poetry Please, Essential Poems*), the poems that have featured in advertising space on London underground trains since 1986 (this project has since been copied around the world in places as diverse as Oslo, St Petersburg, Helsinki and Vienna), and the Poetry Places

'English, which can express the thoughts of Hamlet and the tragedy of King Lear, has no words for the shiver and the headache. The merest schoolgirl, when she falls in love, has Shakespeare or Keats to speak her mind for her, but let a sufferer try to describe a pain in his head to a doctor and language at once runs dry.'
Virginia Woolf, *On Being Ill*

project which has displayed selected poems in public arenas. WB Yeats's poem 'He wishes for the clothes of heaven', which ends with the lines:

> But, I, being poor have only my dreams;
> I have spread my dreams under your feet;
> Tread softly because you tread on my dreams.

was voted the most uplifting poem for people waiting in doctors' receptions.

Does this carry a strong message for healthcare professionals not to forget the vulnerability of patients and the crushing power of 'the white coat'?

HOW DOES POETRY WORK?

RS Thomas attempted an explanation in his poem 'Don't ask me'.

> Don't ask me;
> I have no recipe
> for a poem. You
> know the language,
>
> know where the prose ends
> and poetry begins.
> There should be no
> introit into a poem.
>
> The listener should come
> to and realise
> verse has been going on
> for some time. Let
>
> there be no coughing
> no sighing. Poetry
> is a spell woven'
> by consonants and vowels
>
> in the absence of logic.
> Ask no rhyme
> of a poem, only
> that it keep faith
>
> with life's rhythm.
> Language will trick
> you if it can. Syntax is words'
>
> way of shackling
> the spirit. Poetry is that
> which arrives at the intellect
> by way of the heart.

Poems emphasise imagination, feeling and insight. The text is concentrated, distilling the essence of a feeling, experience or emotion. It may offer comfort in times of distress, but it may just as easily be extremely unsettling. AE Housman said that 'poetry should make your chin hairs bristle with apprehension'. Meaning tends to be implied or inferred rather than spelt out. Poetry finds a way of using words to tell of things and events that we cannot measure, that are difficult to explain and understand. Poems form bridges and make connections between the concrete world in which we live and our inner self. Often this is achieved with the use of image and metaphor.

> I am poured out like water, and all my bones are out of joint: My heart is like wax; it is melted in the midst of my bowels. My strength is dried up like a potsherd.
>
> *Psalm 22*

These statements themselves make no sense. How can a human being be poured out like water? The heart is made of muscle, not wax, and has no direct connection either anatomically or physiologically with the bowels. And yet we all know what the writer of this psalm is talking about. It makes sense as a description of the sensations experienced when in the depths of depression or when seriously physically ill. These are **metaphors** which describe feelings. This psalm is about suffering. The writer is persecuted, frightened and alone. We struggle for words to describe sensations and feelings. We feel 'broken hearted' or 'over the moon' – both unlikely concepts, yet readily understood.

This takes us to the very heart of medical encounters, where we confront and need to try to understand feelings and emotions which are difficult to put into words, and an understanding of poetry might help us with this.

Here is an example in a poem by WH Auden, whose father was a physician. His poem 'Musee des Beaux Arts' tried to explain the image portrayed in Breughel's painting of the fall of Icarus (Icarus is shown falling out of the sky, while a ploughman continues his work without blinking and a luxurious boat continues its voyage without stopping) in terms of the general indifference there is to the suffering that is all around us:

> About suffering they were never wrong,
> The Old Masters: how well they understood
> Its human position; how it takes place
> In Breughels *Icarus*, for instance: how everything turns away
> Quite leisurely from the disaster; the ploughman may

Have heard the splash, the forsaken cry,
But for him it was not an important failure; the sun shone
As it had to on the white legs disappearing into the green
Water; and the expensive delicate ship which must have seen
Something amazing, a boy falling out of the sky,
Had somewhere to get to and sailed calmly on.

Suffering goes on around us all the time, but life with all of its artefacts proceeds relentlessly. Icarus falls out of the sky, a cry or a splash may be heard, but a man continues to plough and a luxury boat sails on apparently indifferent to this catastrophic event. How can this relate to everyday life? A common experience during bereavement is a feeling of detachment from a world which appears oblivious to the desperate plight of the bereaved person, who feels like shouting out 'Hey, stop. Don't you know what has happened to me?'. But the world does not stop, and normal day-to-day activities carry on regardless. Auden is quite brutal in his assessment of human behaviour – he describes 'how everything *turns away quite leisurely* from the disaster'. The catastrophic earth-quake is headline news, but only briefly.

Carole Satyamurti is more explicit with the use of metaphor in her poem, 'Changing the subject', which describes the cancer patient's 'journey' through the hospital system.

Outpatients

Women stripped to the waist,
Wrapped in blue,
We are a uniform edition
Waiting to be read.

These plain covers suit us:
We're inexplicit,
It's not our style to advertise
Our fearful narratives.

My turn. He reads my breasts
Like Braille, finding the lump
I knew was there. This is
the episode I could see coming

– although he's reassuring,
doesn't think its sinister
but just to be quite clear ...
He's taking over,

He'll be the writer now,
The plot master,
And I must wait
To read my next instalment.

In this poem the author reflects on many aspects of the patient's experience, such as the effect of stripping for examination, being intimately examined, and the feeling of being 'taken over' by the surgeon and having her narrative plotted by him. She is able to express them succinctly and imaginatively in language that is rich in metaphor, with dramatic impact, which would have been lost in prose. The poem contains language which questions and challenges our perceptions of reality (*see* the poem 'Disability' later in this chapter). The picture the author paints makes us sit up and think. The images are unsettling; – do we as health professionals really behave like that and create such an experience for our patients?

PRINCIPLES OF WORKING WITH POETRY

We have already discussed in the chapter on 'Teaching with the arts' the importance of having clear aims, achieving engagement with the resource (in this case a poem) and facilitating responses to take the learners into the poet's world and draw correlations with the topic under discussion, whether it be clinical, ethical or some other aspect.

The essential questions to be asked are:

1 What does this poem mean? What is it about?
2 What emotions are expressed?
3 How does it do this?
4 What metaphors are used?
5 What does it make you feel?

You might use Carole Satyamurti's poem for teaching about doctor/ patient interactions and the patient experience, and facilitate with questions such as the following.

- What metaphors are used?
- Are they effective, and if so why?
- What is the significance of the Braille metaphor (e.g. blindness of the surgeon to the whole person)?
- What feelings are generated by the imagery used in the poem?
- Why does the way it is written engage us with the physical dimension of the doctor/patient interaction?

Here is another poem, 'Across the border' by Karen Fiser. It is full of metaphor, which you could use in a similar way to explore the experience of illness:

What are the metaphors used in this poem?

Why are they effective?

Could similar feelings have been so well expressed in prose? If so, how?

For you there was no conscious departure,
no hurried packing for exile
You are here, anyway, in your own
minor archipelago of pain.

Do what every exile does. Tell stories.
Smuggle messages across the border.

Remember the things back there
as simpler than they ever were.

Because of illness (*a journey*), the patient becomes an *exile*, removed from their normal surroundings without preparation. The journey into this foreign country is uncertain. There is a clear boundary (*border*) between past health and current illness. Links with the past state of normal health and explanations are sought in *stories* which themselves are a simplified reconstruction of reality (*see* Chapter 3, 'It's my story', on narrative).

Why are these stories smuggled?

The metaphors have enabled complex feelings and thoughts to be described in simple, easily understood language, using familiar images and analogies.

WORKING WITH WORDS

To learn communication skills, not only must you understand the use of metaphor, but you must also appreciate the power of words themselves. The interpretation of words that patients use is important. Poems are a useful vehicle for this task.

Consider this poem by Emily Dickinson and think about the words she used most effectively to paint a vivid picture of a shaft of winter sunlight.

There's a certain slant of light
On winter afternoons'
That oppresses, like the weight
Of cathedral tunes.

When it comes, the landscape listens,
Shadows hold their breath;
When it goes 'tis like the distance
On the look of death.

The chilling atmosphere is created by the words 'winter', 'weight', 'oppress' and 'shadows', culminating with the image of remoteness from life on the faces of dead people. The phrase 'shadows hold their breath' expresses the double negative feeling of darkness and refusal to breath. A similar feeling might be experienced when listening to parts of Schubert's song cycle *Die Wintereisse* (*see* Chapter 5, 'Sound sense'). We are back in the realm of metaphor. It is resonant with the consultation.

Poems may at first sight not have an obvious meaning – they may need re-reading, reflection and interpretation. We have seen in the poem by Emily Dickinson that they can be usefully studied and analysed in their own right as an exercise to explore how words can convey meaning and feelings.

Can this be translated into our teaching about communication skills in the consultation?

USING POETRY FOR TOPIC TEACHING

When is it appropriate to use poetry? Bereavement and loss, suffering (both physical and mental), social injustice, adolescence and old age, family dysfunction, jealousy and guilt all afflict us and our patients at some time. Many of these themes are explored by poets, and their poems provide some inspirational teaching material.

Here are four examples:

OLD AGE

This is taken from 'The old fools', by Philip Larkin.

> What do they think has happened, the old fools,
> To make them like this? Do they somehow suppose
> It's more grown up when your mouth hangs open and drools,
> And you keep on pissing yourself, and can't remember
> Who called this morning? Or that, if they only chose,
> They could alter things back to when they danced all night,
> Or went to their wedding, or sloped arms some September?
> Or do they fancy there's really been no change,
> And they've always behaved as if they were crippled or tight,
> Or sat through days of thin continuous dreaming
> Watching light move? If they don't (and they can't), its strange:
>   Why aren't they screaming?
>
> Perhaps being old is having lighted rooms
> Inside your head, and people in them, acting.
> People you know, but can't quite name; each looms
> Like a deep loss restored, from known doors turning,
> Setting down a lamp, smailing from a stair, extracting
> A known book from the shelves; or sometimes only
> The rooms themselves, chairs and a fire burning,
> The blown bush at the window, or the sun's
> Faint friendliness on the wallsome lonely
> Rain-ceased midsummer evening. That is where they live:
> Not here and now, but where all happened once.
>   This is why they give

Try asking your learners to analyse a poem of your or their choice. Encourage them to highlight significant words which give the poem direction and meaning. Then ask them to do the same thing with the words used in a consultation, using either a tape recording or a video.

Finally, ask them to write a poem using these words, and metaphors to describe the consultation from either the doctor's or the patient's point of view.

What does this poem teach us about old age, our perception of it and our reaction to it?

Explore perspectives – do we see ourselves in the same way as others do? Does a wounded body make us see others differently?

BODY IMAGE

Here is the poem 'Flower leaning from a vase', by Susan Spady.

One of her breasts
is small and lovely, the other
gone. She practices
asymmetry, flower
leaning from a vase,
rock at the edge
of a bare sill.
She marvels that once
She thought them puny.
Looks with one eye, outward,
inward: does a man with no legs
have spirit
sliced off
like bread?
And does it grow back?
And what of a starving child
whose bones are chalky shadows?

She watches a woman walk home
From church, wig set just so,
Bible clutched to her blank
Chest. What does her body house,
except a dream of perfection?
And what houses the body?
When she filled her babies' bottles
She forced a river
Back into small dry fists.
The doctor advised it.
She traces the mound of fruit
Not picked, and then, her tender
Scar. Could a man stroke this?
And find her?

DISABILITY

Here is the poem 'The handicapped', by Philip Dacey.

How does this poem help us view disability?

1
The missing legs
of the amputee
are somewhere
winning a secret race

2
The blind man has always stood
before an enormous blackboard,
waiting for the first
scrawl of light,
that fine
dusty chalk.

3
Here
the repetitions of the stutterer
there
the flickering
of the stars

4
Master of illusion,
The paralytic alone moves.
All else is still.

5
At Creation,
God told the deaf,
'Only you will hear
the song of the stone.'

6
Dare not ask
what the dumb
have been told to keep secret.

7
When the epileptic
falls in a fit,
he is ascending
to the heaven of earth.

ADOLESCENCE

This is the poem 'Sunglasses', by Sophie Large (written when she was 15 years old).

In an attempt to escape reality
I put on sunglasses,
Because my eyes were dazzled by life.
I grew used to their comforting dimness
And it was only when, many years later,
I remembered I was wearing them,
And found the courage to take them off,
That I realised what I had missed.

> What does this poem teach us about being a teenager?

POETRY AND CREATIVE WRITING SKILLS

The concept of using creative writing to help the understanding of narrative in medicine was introduced in the last chapter. A similar approach can be used when poems are used as a resource, to help learners clarify their insight into the place of poetry and metaphor in comprehending events, and their value as a way of coping with or addressing difficulties.

Write a four-line poem about a current or recent experience as a teacher or medical practitioner which is causing you difficulties and therefore provoking strong feelings and emotions.

The outcome of this exercise has surprised learners.

- Anyone can write a poem.
- The poems are powerful.
- Emotions that were previously buried come to the surface.
- Most learners chose to write about something beyond their control.
- The poems record things that learners were not otherwise able to express.

Here are some examples of poems written by the teachers of general practice:

[Untitled]
He was a big man, everybody said so.
Big in lots of good ways, I mean.
He didn't even diminish in death;
But I felt I did.

[Untitled]
Human needs must be met
Statistics suffocate
The press should scream
Continuity stops dead.

Ten minutes
PMH: Death of a child
The anguish of hope quashed by experience.
Presenting complaint: Fungal nail infection.
The trivia of life carrying on.

[Untitled]
The certainty of the report contrasts with the ambiguity
Of his recent past and soon to be future,
As he gallops unknowingly to passivity;
Protecting me, the voyeuristic stranger within his midst, with his silence.

A big angry patient
Bristling with anger, fit to burst,
Misdirected; not my fault.
So unfair!
So what?

The complaint
The letter arrived
Shockingly, in the mundane pile.
How dare he!
Uncertainty for a while.

These short poems hint at some of the emotions and feelings of experienced doctors working in a time-pressured environment.

There are expressions of anxiety, inadequacy, vulnerability, impotence and (emotional) fatigue – feelings not usually verbalised by health professionals.

Illness and suffering are mysterious, uncomfortable, disturbing and frightening. Poetry, although unable to provide answers, is sometimes able to help with our thinking around and understanding of problems, to put fears and worries into perspective. It helps to articulate disordered thoughts.

The poem 'Punctuation', referred to in Chapter 1, tells us more about the writer's changed life than reams of prose. It has enabled her to express her feelings and work out what the result of the biopsy really means for her as a person, and not just as a patient with a particular diagnosis.

Could it be helpful to have a repertoire of poems to share with patients at these times? Would they be more helpful than a sedative or antidepressant? This is an argument to share with your learners.

POETRY IN TIMES OF CRISIS

These examples explore a further use of poetry in medical education, namely poetry in personal development, as a vehicle to begin to express feelings (hurt, etc.) felt by many health professionals and by patients (already touched upon in the section on creative poetry writing). Poetry begins to give insight into crises (however large or small), to describe them, to give them some narrative coherence and to contain them. As we have seen above, it also gives an outlet for expressing them.

People often to turn to poetry at life's turning points and at times of crisis. Even the loss of an argument can lead to deep-felt regrets which need an outlet. Consider this extract from a poem by Conrad Aiken.

The Quarrel
Suddenly, after the quarrel, while we waited,
Disheartened, silent, with downcast looks, nor stirred
Eyelid nor finger, hopeless both, yet hoping
Against all hope to unsay the sundered word: …

How often have we felt like that after an argument, and how comforting it is to have a common emotion so eloquently expressed.

If you can find resonance with a poem in these circumstances, even though written by someone else, it can articulate in a very concentrated and permanent way your deep thoughts and feelings. It can bring comfort and resolution.

EPILOGUE

Poems, like narratives, are a fund of teaching material. They stimulate the imagination in the quest for meanings, they are a means of looking sideways at the commonplace with metaphor and they are a vehicle for self expression.

However, words are sometimes inadequate. TS Eliot explored their ephemeral nature in this extract from his poem 'Burnt Norton'.

> … Words strain,
> Crack and sometimes break, under the burden,
> Under the tension, slip, slide, perish,
> Decay with imprecision, will not stay in place,
> Will not stay still. Shrieking voices
> Scolding, mocking, or merely chattering,
> Always assail them.

What medium is therefore left to explore human emotions and feelings – the essence of what it means to be human? The next chapter will look at the ability of music to do this.

REFERENCES

Aiken C (2004) The quarrel. In: N Astley (ed.) *Staying Alive*. Bloodaxe Books, Tarset.

Auden WH (1948) Musee Des Beaux Arts. In: J Bayley (ed.) *Good Companions*. Abacus, London.

Dacey P (1991) The handicapped. In: L Dittrich (ed.) *Ten Years of Medicine and the Arts*. Academic Medicine, Washington, DC.

Dickinson E (1951) There's a certain slant of light. In: S Heaney and T Hughes (eds) *The Rattle Bag*. Faber & Faber, London.

Eliot TS (1936) *Four Quartets: Burnt Norton*. In: *Collected Poems 1909–1962*. Faber & Faber, London.

Fiser K (1992) Across the border. In: *Words Like Fate and Pain*. Steerforth Press, Hanover, NH.

Large S (1998) Sunglasses. In: *Sophie's Log*. Sophie's Silver Lining Fund, Banbury.

Larkin P (1974) The old fools. In: *High Windows*. Faber and Faber, London.

Satyamurti C (2000) Outpatients. In: N Astley (ed.) *Staying Alive*. Bloodaxe Books, Tarset.

Spady S (2001) Flower leaning from a vase. In: L Dittrich (ed.) *Ten Years of Medicine and the Arts*. Academic Medicine, Washington, DC.

Thomas RS (2002) Don't ask me. In: M Wynn Thomas (ed.) *Residues*. Bloodaxe Books, Tarset.

Woolf V (2002) *On Being Ill*. Paris Press, Ashfield, MA.

5 SOUND SENSE

Throughout this book we emphasise the value of the creative arts in facilitating engagement with the human aspect of medicine – understanding patients' experiences, emotions and feelings, and developing empathy. The juxtaposition of art and medical science allows doctors their own humanity and lets them feel those emotions that their patients experience. In the previous chapter, about poetry, we looked at the way in which poems expressed feelings through words. Music can powerfully express how we feel. It can be resonant with our mood and help others to understand and communicate those feelings through non-verbal language. Consider how music can enhance visual and verbal images in films. For example, *Nessun Dorma* from Puccini's opera *Turandot* is used in the film *The Killing Fields*, in which the character Sydney Schanberg comes back to New York from Cambodia, desperately worried about his friend Dith Pran, whom he has left behind. He spends hours watching and searching TV film footage of the war in that country in the hope of seeing him. The emotional impact of this scene is extraordinarily heightened by the accompanying music, which provides the emotional background, and allows us to draw even more from this moment of drama.

To engage with music we must listen and interpret, and during interpretation of the sound we hear we must use our imagination. These are very similar to the skills that we require to be transported into patients' lives when we try to understand their problems, and therefore exercises built around a musical resource can be powerful teaching tools. In this chapter we look at a variety of ways in which music can be harnessed to help us understand the experience of being a patient:

'Only when I experience do I compose – only when I compose do I experience.'
Gustav Mahler (1860–1911)

1   to enhance listening skills
2   to enhance interpretive skills and encourage imaginative thinking
3   to promote emotional awareness
4   to give an insight into the nature of suffering
5   to engage learners in the experience of illness through the drama of opera and ballet.

LISTENING SKILLS

Listening is one of the primary skills employed during patient encounters.

> Listen to the slow movement of Beethoven's fourth piano concerto and ask your learners to describe what is happening in this piece of music. What are they hearing? Emphasise that you do not need to be a musician to complete this task. This is not a question of music appreciation.

The music is a dialogue between the piano and the strings of the orchestra. At first the piano is quiet, muted and reticent, and the strings are loud, firm and dominant. As the dialogue progresses the roles are reversed – the strings become quiet and the piano becomes gradually louder and more strident. When facilitating this exercise, concentrate on simple things such as the pitch, volume and rhythm of the music, and the relationship of the piano to the rest of the orchestra.

There are plenty of other examples of 'dialogues' in music. For example, much jazz is constructed around relationships between instruments.

> Listen to the second movement of Mozart's Symphony No. 40 and look out for the 'conversation' between instruments in different parts of the orchestra.

Some learners might question the validity of using music for this sort of exercise in listening skills. Why not use consultation videos or simulated patients? We would suggest that music adds another dimension – it is another way of looking at a familiar scenario (this is discussed further in Chapter 6, 'A way of seeing').

INTERPRETATION AND IMAGINATION

In Chapter 3 on narrative medicine we discussed the way in which *we* construct a narrative when a patient tells us *their* story. We think laterally – we use our imagination. Music is a useful tool for developing these skills. We are using music as a narrative vehicle. The exercises are a natural progression from the listening exercises described above to an interpretation of what we are hearing. It is not just a plain narrative we hear, but a story in which moods are expressed. We want our learners to be aware of this when they communicate with patients.

> Listen again to the slow movement of Beethoven's fourth piano concerto. Having established what is happening within the music, ask your learners to construct a narrative from it. What story is being told in this musical dialogue? Not only does this exercise promote listening skills, but it also stimulates the use of the imagination.

'Are we hearing an argument?', 'Is there a battle going on?' (or could it be a consultation?).

Listening to the first movement of the Brahms violin concerto provoked the following interpretive responses.

- 'There is a build up of tension and expectation.'
- 'Tension resolved as peace.'
- 'Listening to the music was like standing on the brink.'
- 'It was precipitous.'
- 'It was like water falling.'

Many composers of all types of music have composed music which does deliberately attempt to tell a story (programme music) or interpret a story (e.g. opera, lieder, folk song, blues, film music, blues and spirituals).

> This could be illustrated by using *The March to the Scaffold* from *Symphonie Fantastique* by Berlioz. Ask your learners to construct the narrative from this music (a poet has killed his beloved and is being marched to the gallows – the ugliness of the occasion is stressed by raucous brass instruments).

Opera is good resource to use here to explore your learners' powers of interpretation and imagination, as you can play the music, facilitate the interpretation and then show a video or DVD of the same passage to show the original narrative.

We have used the end of Act 2 of Puccini's *Tosca*, a graphic picture of mental abuse and torture, as an exercise.

Songs are a rich source of narrative.

Der Leiermann, in Schubert's introspective song cycle *Wintereisse*, atmospherically portrays the wanderer (possibly the composer himself, who knew that he was suffering from syphilis and probably facing a terminal illness with dementia and paralysis) pondering his perceived hopeless fate.

Your own list of music (not necessarily classical in origin) could be used in a similar way.

EMOTIONAL AWARENESS

Listen to the Cavatina from Beethoven's string quartet opus 130. What do you *feel* after hearing it? What emotions did you experience? What other pieces of music do you know from any genre which have the same effect?

The emotional impact on many people of this piece of music by Beethoven is profound. There is deep pain and sadness, and an agonizing cry for relief, for happiness and peace, which do not come. The sorrowful and bitter opening is followed by the second theme which Beethoven scores to be played *Beklemmt* (anguished). There is real agony here. Could it perhaps be the anguish of grief?

Beethoven considered this movement to be the crowning achievement of his chamber music, a sentiment echoed by many musicians and reflected in the decision to put a recording of it in the *Voyager* spacecraft.

How can listening to music like this help medical practitioners? What relevance does it have to everyday life within the medical context?

Much professional time is spent with patients who are confronting pain, disability, depression and death, and trying to cope with a range of mostly negative emotions (e.g. sorrow and sadness, anger, frustration, fear, shock, loneliness, despair, rejection and alienation, disappointment, and pessimism). Mercifully, there are sometimes positive emotions to be recognised and shared (e.g. hope, relief and joy).

When we listen to the patient's narrative, we are hearing not only words but also the expression of these very feelings. As medical professionals we must be able to be 'in tune' and recognise these feelings, both in our patients and in ourselves. It is part of the process of developing empathy with and understanding of our patients and self-awareness in ourselves. The concept of *emotional intelligence* (self-awareness, managing emotions, self-motivation, empathy and interpersonal effectiveness), first described by Aristotle in 350 BC, is now being recognised as an important component of professional development. Listening to music with a high emotional content can be a means of developing this ability.

> Ask your learners to bring a piece of music which for them has high emotional content, with an explanation of what that particular piece means to them and why. The place of emotional response can then be explored with a group.

A great variety of music is usually produced in response to this exercise, from Mozart to the latest chart-topping piece of pop music.

A Mozart wind serenade was felt to portray 'aching and wistful longing with no resolution to hope'. A piece of new world music was described as 'peaceful and tranquil'.

The appreciation of music is very subjective. A piece of music may induce different reactions in different people. This is worth exploring and discussing in order to tease out the nature of emotional response. Why do certain people respond in a certain way to a given stimulus? This response may not necessarily occur every time a particular piece of music is played. It may depend on the listener's underlying emotional state at that time. Does this give any insight into our needs as health professionals? Can we be trained to be more emotionally aware?

Another way of looking at this is demonstrated by the next exercise:

> Ask your learners to list the emotions that their patients may exhibit and then to match them with pieces of music which give expression to similar feelings. Emphasise that all types of music – classical, pop, jazz, soul, etc. – are equally valid.

We considered in the introduction to this chapter how music has been used to create 'moods' or paint an emotional background in films. This exercise is another 'way in' for discussing emotional intelligence.

> Show your learners an extract from the film *Brief Encounter* and ask them why the music (Rachmaninov's second piano concerto) is so effective in enhancing the emotional effect of the dialogue.

Beware: You may have people in your learners' group for whom music means nothing – this a facilitator's challenge. Be prepared to cope with such negative feelings about an exercise (*see* Chapter 2, 'Teaching with the arts', Feedback).

THE NATURE OF SUFFERING

We have said earlier that music may be able to express suffering when our vocabulary does not contain adequate words to do so.

> Ask your learners to describe any music which for them depicts pain or suffering.

Many of the great classical composers themselves experienced chronic debilitating physical illness during their lifetime (Beethoven was profoundly deaf and had cirrhosis, Schubert had syphilis, Mahler suffered from rheumatic heart disease resulting in atrial fibrillation and considerable hypochondriasis, Smetana had syphilis which resulted in dementia). Some are thought to have had psychiatric problems, in particular bipolar affective disorder. Could this have had an impact on their creativity and the music they composed? Is the composer able to express his or her innermost feelings in a way that words fail to do? Is it helpful for us to understand this insight into the nature of suffering?

The composer Robert Schumann had a depressive illness associated with auditory hallucinations. He sometimes heard voices urging him to compose.

> Listen to *Kreisleriana*. Does Schumann give any hint here of mental anguish, and of the psychotic symptoms which would eventually lead him to attempt suicide.

Mozart, who is thought by some to have had a bipolar disorder, composed his last three symphonies (Nos 39, 40 and 41) in the space of only a few weeks, but at a time of personal desperation.

> Play the *Andante Cantabile* (second movement) from Mozart's *Symphony No. 41*. Does this give any hint of his mental state?

The Czech composer Bedrich Smetana composed his second string quartet in a lunatic asylum while suffering from tertiary syphilis and, like Schumann, experiencing disturbing auditory hallucinations and loss of ability to remember melodies.

> Is Smetana's condition expressed in his music? Does it help us to understand his feelings? Are there any pointers to what it feels like to suffer? Is this an insight into what it feels like to be a patient? Is it possible, through music, to experience what your patient is going through?

THE EXPERIENCE OF ILLNESS IN OPERA

Opera is a powerful art form, combining music, drama and narrative. We see, we hear and we experience emotion when we are at the opera.

Many operas are concerned with themes of illness and mortality, and through them composers have often set disease within social contexts and stereotypes (e.g. women have tuberculosis (TB) and are responsible for its transmission – the tubercular female was portrayed as desired, desirable and desiring; men have syphilis, having been infected by women).

Here are some ideas for the use of opera as a teaching resource in clinical medicine:

TB

The classic TB operas are *La Boheme* by Puccini and *La Traviata* by Verdi, and these can usefully be utilised to study the effect of illness on the individual and those around them, and its effect on relationships and attitudes. Both heroines die on stage, and this portrayal of their death could be used in discussions about terminal care and dying.

CHILD ABUSE

Peter Grimes by Benjamin Britten is the grim story of child abuse by a loner and an outcast in a close-knit and suspicious community – powerful themes which are ripe for discussion.

SMOKING

Carmen by Bizet is the story of a beautiful but wilful woman, soldiers, a toreador, and passionate love with a tragic ending. At the start it is set around a cigarette factory and cigarettes and smoking are an integral ingredient of the early part of the opera. Could this enhance a session on smoking cessation and broaden thinking on issues around the symbolism of smoking (*see* Chapter 6, 'A way of seeing').

SUICIDE

There is death by suicide in several operas. *Madame Butterfly* by Puccini is the poignant story of a Japanese geisha who, against the cultural wishes of her family, 'marries' an itinerant US sailor, and after a long wait for his return discovers that he has married an American wife. She stabs herself on stage, leaving her 4-year old son.

In all these examples music has been used to enhance an educational experience. It has been a 'way in'. It has been a different way of looking at common topics, and has provided the catalyst for discussion.

FINAL ACT

Music is one of the more difficult of the creative arts to work with in medical education. It is abstract and learners may be put off by the perceived exclusivity of classical music and media such as opera.

'Will my Bob Dylan be too low brow? To my surprise it struck a chord!'

The examples cited in this chapter *are* mostly from classical music, but other styles of music, and music from all cultures, are equally valid for this type of work. The actual choice of music rests with the facilitator and the learners, but the aims of using music must be made clear and explicit from the outset.

We have seen above how music can paint pictures. Music has even been written to 'illustrate' and accompany paintings (e.g. Mussorgsky's *Pictures at an Exhibition*). The next chapter looks at the use of visual images as a resource.

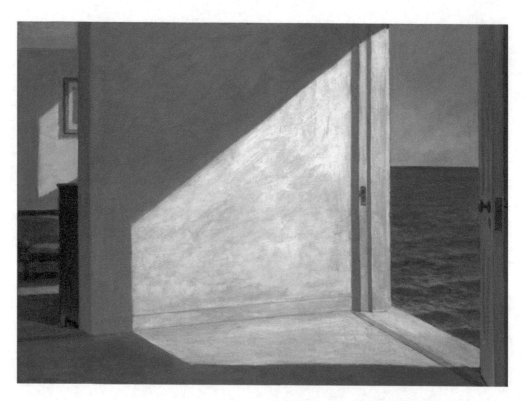

Figure 6.1 *Rooms by the Sea* (1951), by Edward Hopper

6 A WAY OF SEEING

INTRODUCTION

VISUAL THINKING

When patients try to describe events and how they felt at the time, they set scenes, and in doing so they use their own imagery. In listening to their descriptions, you in turn form pictures in your own mind. You hear the narrative and see the context.

This is visual thinking, and it is an essential part of the communication process.

The pictures you form, and the images that are given by the patient, are important pieces of information which aid your understanding and interpretation of the patient's needs.

Visual thinking also means being able to see what is happening *in front* of you, or being able to pick up visual cues and clues. It's a skill to be able to catch those fleeting impressions of patients that yield so much about them and freeze the frame, the stilled narrative.

All this is what we do to some extent most of the time in daily life. What follows in this discussion of using the art resource is aimed at enhancing and sharpening awareness of this natural process.

Each moment passes fleetingly, so using images which have been made permanent by the artist gives us time to examine similar moments in detail. Artists observe, capture and record. In addition, they can express the essence of things. So this is why we suggest engaging with art as a way of allowing the examination of moments in a wide range of human activity. It will increase the store of information about such moments, which will in turn help us hold on to and to understand our own impressions. It exercises observational skills, interpretation of what we see and what it can make us feel, and how that can influence subsequent action and decision-making.

'Thanks to Art, instead of seeing one world, our own, we see it multiplied and as many original artists as there are, so many worlds are at our disposal.'
Marcel Proust (1871–1922)

WHAT IS ART?

Attempts to state philosophically what art is do not lead to any straightforward definition. Art may have a function in expressing emotion or in stimulating aesthetic pleasure. Its context, how it is created and what it seeks to show may be relevant as a way of drawing attention to themes and attitudes of the time. A little like genetic material on a chromosome, it may have the ability to express traits, to define all those handed-down experiences in human history and to prompt recognition for the viewer in their own life. For example, if you look at medieval fresco painting on the walls of a country Italian church, the features of the faces are the same as those of the villagers you have just walked past, and the portrayal of joy and distress in the demeanour and stance of the people in the painting is identifiable with those patients you have seen in your work.

So with regard to visual art, a created visual or tactile piece of work, it is how you *react* to it that probably defines it as such, fulfilling some of the above criteria. This means that you can dislike, as well as like, a piece of art you see, just as you may have differing feelings about every person you meet, when you look at them. What is important is to think about what you are seeing, and to seek ways of extending your vision and perceptions. Remember that everything in the intellect has started from the senses and their input.

There can be a joy, fascination, excitement, aesthetic pleasure in looking at art. In some way this can stimulate, calm, stir the imagination, intrigue, widen your view, or add interest to the day, as the creativity of the artist is transferred to the viewer. It can make you feel good, and relax you.

Looking at art may be a new experience. Groups talking about pictures become animated and absorbed, wanting to share their ideas and responses – something happens, always. It is possible to start the process of engaging with art from *any* response.

'Art teaches nothing, except the significance of life.'

Henry Miller

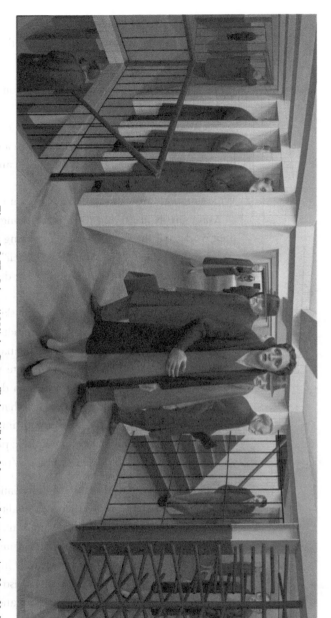

Figure 6.2 *The Subway* (1950), by George Tooker. Whitney Museum of American Art, New York. Purchased with funds from the Juliana Force Purchase Award 50.23

USING ART IMAGES IN TEACHING

In the examples and discussion that follows, three questions form the basis for using art as a resource:

1 What is in the art work that can tell you something about people?

   For example, art as a visual narrative can show scenes of social reality and relationships, and can catch the essence of infirmity, old age, childhood or illness. It can show the human body in all its forms and actions.

2 What emotions are expressed? How does it make you feel?

   Many artists are trying to express feelings and thoughts in their works, but there is little value in staying with the questions 'What did *they* mean?' or 'What did *they* feel?'. For our purposes it is better to stick with the question 'What do *I* see?', 'What do *I* feel?' and 'What do *I* respond to?'.

3 How can art work be used to practise the skill of observation?

   Observation means looking in detail, not just scanning. For example, in the consultation there may be many different minor shifts in the face and eyes, which indicate the patient's state of mind. So exercises that ask learners to describe everything they can see in a picture, and to justify what it is they see that informs their interpretation, will help to improve their ability when examining patients to get the holistic picture, rather than seeing only a particular piece of anatomy/pathology.

It is not our intention to undertake art appreciation (i.e. an analysis of the painting, its style, significance and quality), but, as stressed earlier, to reflect on how the art affects and informs you and thus contributes to your knowledge about yourself and others. We have found that using paintings and photographs in group work with the aim of considering the above questions also acts as a stimulus, a catalyst, a touchpaper for the imagination, and for discussion of important issues in life.

   The process of expressing what is within a painting is exemplified and extended in further ways. The poet translates the essence of the painting into words (*see* WH Auden's poem about Breughel's painting *The Fall of Icarus* in Chapter 4, at page 47), which in their turn may sharpen awareness and understanding of the painting, as the poet shares his or her insight and feelings engendered by it. Similarly, the composer depicts in music his or her understanding of the mood of the paintings, as Mussorgsky did with his work *Pictures at an Exhibition*.

THINGS YOU CAN DO AS TASKS AND EXERCISES

A good place to start, where there are readily available paintings to look at, is a public art gallery or museum.

VISITING ART GALLERIES AND MUSEUMS

Individual visits

Examples of responses

- 'I've seen a David Hockney painting at Saltaire Mill [Figure 6.3]. It's a commissioned portrait of a married couple and their cat.'
- 'It made me wonder about them, the way he shows them sitting totally apart. The window going right down the middle of the painting divides them too.'

Facilitation can encourage learners to elaborate further on what they saw and felt, and how this may tell them something about the relationship. Ask if it connects with anything they have seen or felt about patients.

Draw attention to the learner's sense of curiosity – wanting to know more, being drawn into the narrative of the painting. Why?

Learners are asked to go on their own to an art gallery or museum of their choice. They are asked to make notes on one exhibit that draws their attention and to acquire a postcard or catalogue photo of it if possible, to bring to the group. Then work in small groups of four to six people. In turn, each group member presents their chosen art work, and explains why they chose it, what it did for them and what they saw. As each presentation is mad, the facilitator encourages comments and responses from other group members and discussion about issues that arise.

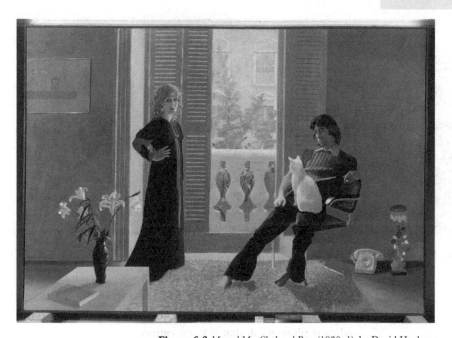

Figure 6.3 *Mr and Mrs Clark and Percy* (1970–1), by David Hockney

Another member of a group said this:

- 'I chose a Lowry picture of people going into the factory where they work. I think it connects for me about my own inner city Practice, and why I chose to do that kind of work. He's made those people like the ones I know.'

The facilitator can get the learner to illustrate in more detail from the picture what all the characters are doing, how they are grouped and depicted, and to pursue his or her statement about the choice of work. Why is affirmation important? The learner can also reflect about the significance of recognition, offering understanding and initiating empathy. Encourage the group to contribute their experiences of this.

- 'This is a photograph of Wasdale Head in the Lake District in Cumbria. I've got it on my consulting room wall now too. It gives me great happiness, because when I'm walking there I feel good and I want to hold onto that.'

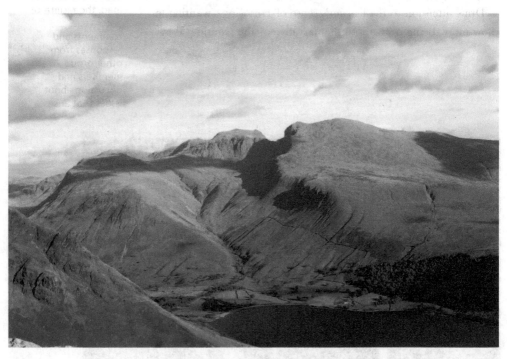

Figure 6.4 Wasdale Head, Cumbria

The facilitator can use this statement to illustrate how an image can act as a way back into an emotion, to reinforce something that has been experienced and that can be reapplied in another situation. Ask the learner to show the other group members what it is in the landscape photograph that is so evocative.

Group visits

Going in a group means that participants can share their thoughts, feelings and intuitions as they experience them. This may spark off other responses, and they may learn from each other.

You can go to an art gallery as part of any teaching, to promote the concept that learning can be effective in *any* situation. Consider that the aim of the visit is to examine response and understanding. The situation in this case is an art gallery, but it is unusual, atypical and unlike traditional medical education venues. In common with environments where medical care may be needed, it shows aspects of human activity and emotions. Thus doing this exercise can help to prepare medical personnel for the many different events in their jobs where they will *have* to be able to respond effectively and remain equable when presented with the unfamiliar, the perhaps apparently chaotic, or the unpredictable.

An exhibition at a gallery may have a theme which links with other work you are doing with a group. It will be an additional resource for learning

Practical point

Visit the exhibition yourself beforehand, so that you know what is there, its size and layout. This will enable you to plan how much time you will need to get there and look around the exhibition, what instructions (if any) to give learners, and where the café is!

Example of a group visit exercise

We went to an exhibition of work by Terry Atkinson at Leeds City Art Gallery entitled 'Confrontation and Continuation'. There were strong images, both *figurative* and *abstract*, of the social reality of contemporary war, with an emphasis on conflict, futility and the fragility of human values. It linked with the work we had already done with narrative, in considering *Regeneration* by Pat Barker (*see* page 34).

Here we considered the impact of visual images in expressing conflict and our responses to this. There was a curiosity about trying to understand things represented in a different way. The group agreed that having, as a given task, really to look in detail at the art work, to think about their reactions, to enquire of each other's responses, and to be generous in engaging with the facilitator's venture and give it a go, meant that although they might not have 'liked' or 'agreed with' all of the artist's work, it had certainly made them examine some of their own areas of comfort, prejudice, denial and comprehension.

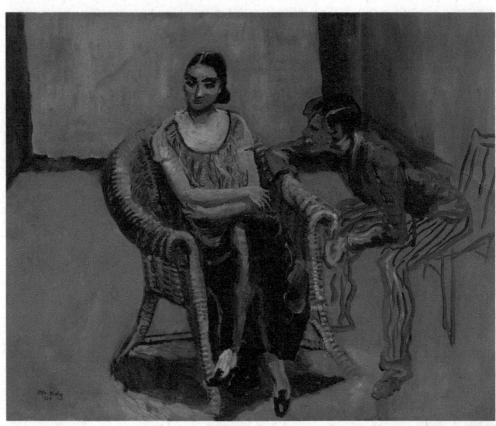

Figure 6.5 *A Couple* (1925), by Per Krog.
Lillehammer Art Museum
(Photo: Jacques Lathion)

> Show the painting in Figure 6.5 to a small group, on a screen.
>
> The people in the painting are the next patients who have come into the consulting room. Take time to look at them.
>
> How will you start this consultation? What have you already seen and surmised?
>
> How does it affect what you will do next? What responses will you need to be aware of?

What happens

Learners can pick up the body language in the painting – the women's arms across her chest as a barrier and holding herself together, her head turned away, and the attempt by the man to engage with her, leaning forward, braced, and trying to get her attention. How can the doctor make contact with her as well?

Learners can debate the narrative of this couple's relationship. Which one is the patient, or is it both of them? What is going on that is indicated by the way the artist has shown them, apparently in discord.

Learners can try out phrases and words to use when speaking to the couple, while the facilitator encourages discussion about effectiveness and choice – for example, the value of the open statement and reflection 'You look troubled ...' in indicating empathy.

This exercise connects the parts of the process of communication.

- What do I see and feel?
- Why is it affecting me?
- How can I respond effectively?

What is the point of using a painting or photograph like this, instead of simulated patients or role play with a real person?

It's a good way of gradually getting people going, perhaps at the beginning of communication skills training. The image is fixed, it won't change, and there's plenty of time to absorb, think and talk about it before starting to take any action. It is a common focus for the whole group, so that when someone says 'I think I'd say to her ...' it is less threatening than one-to-one role play, or conducting a consultation with a simulator in front of everyone. It has become an extended part of the discussion.

It is good to follow up this type of exercise with living 'patients' and have things to try that have been practised and are thus more familiar.

COMMUNICATING WITH CHILDREN

Think about books for young children. The narrative is always enhanced by pictures.

- What do the pictures succeed in communicating? How do children respond?
- How are children depicted in art? What aspects of their activity and demeanour are heightened?
- How can considering these things help become better at being with children?

Tasks

1 Look at a painting showing children involved in some activity, such as *Children Port Glasgow* by Joan Eardley. This painting can be found in Duncan MacMillan's book *Scottish Art*, but for copyright reasons it is not reproduced here. It is a painting that graphically shows the relationships of children to each other, and the tension between play and the need to take on a more adult role when an older child is responsible for a younger one. Ask the group to think about what they see and feel. What sort of things could they talk about with the children?

2 Look at children's books. Think about how the stories are told in words and pictures. What seem to be the authors' aims? Have they got it right? Examples of books you might use are *Mr Bump* by Roger Hargreaves and books illustrated by Quentin Blake.

To communicate effectively with children it is necessary to have the ability to listen and tune in to a child's world. It may mean bypassing the developed, rational adult mind and entering again into playfulness, being creative, and calling back the child within you – your own memories and experiences. When participants are given the above resources, they have the licence to respond as if they were children – they can play around, engaging with Mr Bump. They remember being together with other kids, like the Glasgow children, and start talking about it. You could use some of the drama work with 'playing' (*see* Chapter 9, 'The drama of everyday life') during the same session.

USING ART RESOURCES FOR TOPIC TEACHING IN THE MEDICAL CURRICULUM

The learner not only needs biological knowledge about an illness and its effects, but also needs to comprehend the *experience for the patient* of that illness and their beliefs and expectations. It is here that art can be a useful resource.

Here are some examples of the use of the art resource in teaching about **eating disorders**, **women's health** and **smoking cessation**.

Eating disorders

What are the concepts that are important in understanding and managing these disorders? The following exercise starts the process of thinking about perceptions of body image and shape.

Jenny Saville's painting *Branded* (Figure 6.6) labels and reinforces obesity through the subject pinching up her skinfold ('Look at me, I'm fat'), but her head is drawn back, almost in retreat. Learners consider and talk about the image. This can focus their thinking and hopefully engage their attention. It is a good preparation

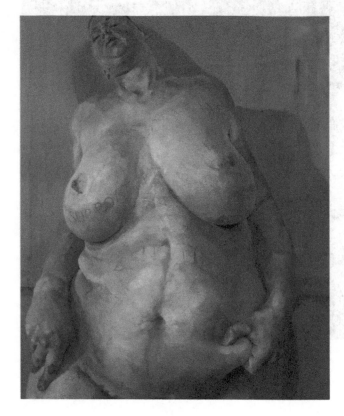

Figure 6.6 *Branded* (1992), by Jenny Saville

before moving on to teaching diagnosis and treatment of disorders. It can start an element of enquiry and interest, which displaces the learner's feelings of being overwhelmed, and of incomprehension ('This is something I just don't understand'), when confronted with, for example, an anorexic patient. It can also help people think about their own ideas about their bodies.

Women's health

Successful management results from including the patient as an equal participant in decision-making, and so we need to know about, and be aware of, things that will influence this discussion with regard to her health, namely:

- her emotions
- dilemmas associated with her social and personal life
- hidden fears and anxieties.

Images of women in painting and photography can capture and record some of this. Here is an example (Figure 6.7).

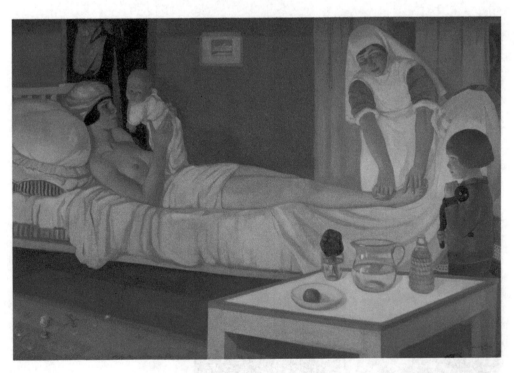

Figure 6.7 *Romance* (1921), by Cecile Walton

1 Look at the response of the mother to her new baby. She is holding the baby away from her, an expression of puzzlement and
uncertainty on her face. The baby is not looking at the mother.
Perhaps there is denial/rejection by the mother, and maybe the
beginnings of depression?
2 Observe the nurse/carer who is washing the patient. She is
looking only at what she is doing, and appears distant from the
mother, certainly not communicating with her. This emphasises
the mother's isolation.
3 Note how the child clutches tightly to her doll's leg. She is
very removed from the mother and almost out of the picture,
perhaps metaphorically, as if excluded, the new baby taking
her place, and the mother not seeming able to draw her into
her affection.
4 The title *Romance* suggests a note of cynicism. Note the discarded
flower on the floor, the petals scattered. There is no happy father
in the painting.

Although this painting was done in 1921 and practices have
changed with regard to care after childbirth, it retains universal
experiences, as described above, which are still relevant today.
Teaching with this painting as a focus could include recognising
the early signs of puerperal depression, the role of carers, and the
behaviour of siblings and their needs. So the painting:

• depicts a narrative about a human event with identifiable
characters
• can spark off questions about the demeanour of the characters,
which leads to an analysis of feelings towards and about them
• contains much information in its details, For example, did you
notice the scattered petals on the floor, when you first *glanced* at
the painting?

In teaching about women's health, the use of paintings depicting
women can be effective in multidisciplinary groups (midwives,
doctors, clinic staff). Here the images represent a common interest
regardless of individual staff viewpoints.

The lecturer can create a narrative with pictures that show
'patients'. The visual impact engages learners, perhaps more than
a written slide would do. It will connect and remind them of
scenarios from their own professional experience, and it will create
links.

You could use the learners' responses to this in subsequent small group work. For example, you could see how each group member responded to a painting, what they picked out about the woman and how this might differ for each depending on their job, thus enabling a sharing of insights not only about the patient but also about their own roles.

Smoking cessation

Smoking is something that doctors have to deal with. In general, they have to give information about the health risks and help people to give up smoking if they want to do so. In particular, when people come with an illness that is clearly smoking-related, doctors have to let them know this. The question is how to go about it.

Consider the principles involved in behavioural support techniques for stopping smoking. They involve understanding the patient's history and their motivation, identifying situations where they most want to smoke, and thinking about coping strategies to deal with this. Thus the doctor needs to be sensitive to the whole person, and be able to empathise, and not be blinkered or stuck in the tramline of just *telling* people what they should or should not do.

The kinds of paintings/photographs (where people are smoking) to look for and use are those in which the artist has caught something more about that person than we might notice in just passing by. Looking at such a painting stimulates discussion about our experience both of ourselves and of others as prompted by what we see in it. There is time to contemplate such a fixed image and reflect, to engage with the person, and to start to learn the dialogue that encompasses that person's world and their own ideas and beliefs.

Questions you could use to invite responses might include the following.

- What do you know about this person from their stance, features and expression?
- What do you feel about them?
- How could you talk to them about their life?

In this self-portrait by Edvard Munch (Figure 6.8, opposite), painted when he was 28 years old, he chooses an image of himself that incorporates the cigarette. We know that he was an artist who suffered from anxiety and depression, his famous work *The Scream* depicting much of the despair of mental illness. He captures and records a lot of himself in this image, the cigarette

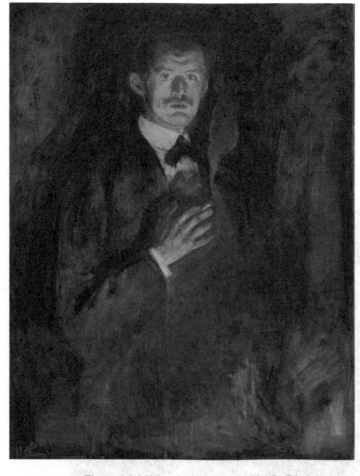

Figure 6.8 *Self Portrait with a Cigarette* (1895), by Edward Munch.
National Gallery, Norway. © 2004 Munch Museum/Munch-Ellingsen Group,
BONO, Oslo and DACS, London

held prominently across his chest in the centre of the painting,
its whiteness a contrast to the sombre colours of his clothes and
background, ensuring that it is noticed.

USING PAINTINGS/PHOTOGRAPHS THAT SHOW STATES OF ILLNESS

A medical textbook can give factual information about the signs
and symptoms of a disease, often accompanied by isolated close-up
photographs of lesions, rashes, etc. What the artist can do in a
painting that shows an ill person is to capture the real feeling of that
illness, what it means for the patient, what they are experiencing
and how their body is responding.

Last Sickness (Figure 6.9) is a portrait of the artist's mother. She fell, fractured her hip and failed to recover as complications set in. Alice Neel captures the weariness and resignation of her mother, the sadness of the eyes, the thin pursed mouth, the slump of her posture. We can see she is inwardly suffering, as well as enduring illness.

Good clinical judgement means combining scientific knowledge with a humane attitude, empathy and understanding. Giving learners the opportunities to look at such paintings means they

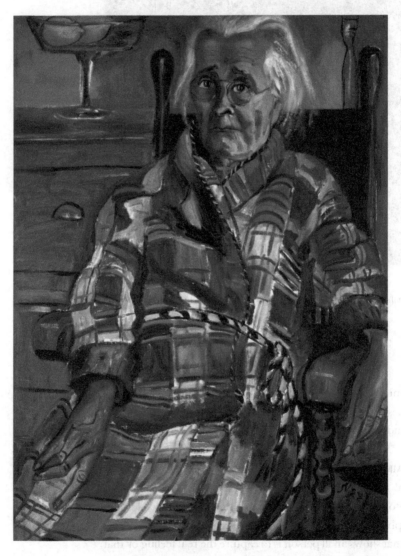

Figure 6.9 *Last Sickness* (1953), by Alice Neel. © Estate of Alice Neel.
Courtesy of Robert Miller Gallery, New York

can reflect on what they see and gain insight. When learners apply such insights to their work, the patient becomes a whole person to whom they can relate, and not just some isolated pathology that has to be dealt with.

OTHER IDEAS

Use photographs of sculptures (classical and modern) which depict the human body to look at posture and anatomy relevant to medical conditions which affect the back. How do people stand and move? What is normal? How can you recognise abnormality?

We have illustrated our ideas in this chapter with art taken from Europe and North America – in other words, Western Art, the culture with which we are most familiar. There is a huge resource of art from other world cultures, and we are aware of the need to extend our knowledge of it, so that we can start to include some. It would be excellent in a diverse group of learners to encourage group members to present art from their own cultures, to look at the responses and discuss how this art is relevant to aspects of that culture in promoting understanding.

We used a series of paintings and photographs as a PowerPoint presentation without commentary, showing images of people that illustrated ethnicity, gender, family life, modes of dress, age and relationships, as a start to a one-day workshop entitled 'Working with Diversity'. The intention of the day was to enable participants to understand themselves, colleagues and patients better, by examining attitudes to cultural diversity and developing ideas about the nature of diversity, ethnicity and culture, and to feel more confident as GPs working with a diverse range of patient populations. The images were effective in engaging learners in thinking widely and starting to reflect on the topic before moving into group work.

So try some of the exercises in this chapter, or devise your own. In the next chapter we shall go out on location, to see the world and look at art in a wider context.

FURTHER READING

The Art Book (1994) and *The Twentieth Century Art Book*. Phaidon, London.

Each has 500 pictures of works of art, with short commentaries, not just about the artist, but also about the context and the significance of the work, so they are useful source books, and available in a pocket size as well as a larger format.

de Botton A (2002) *The Art Of Travel*. Penguin, Harmondsworth.
    Debates how and what we see, with examples from art, in an
    entertaining style and encompassing philosophical ideas.
Warburton N (2003) *The Art Question*. Routledge, London.
    'A stimulating and handy guide through the art maze … essential
    reading for those who simply like looking at and thinking about
    pictures.'

7 OUT ON LOCATION

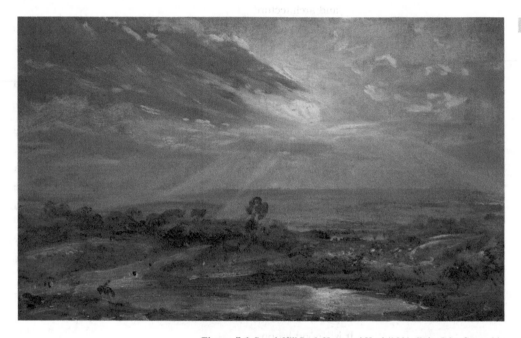

Figure 7.1 *Branch Hill Pond, Hampstead Heath* (1821–2), by John Constable

USING THE WORLD IN MEDICAL EDUCATION

'Who saw the narrow sunbeam that came out of the south, and
smote upon their summits until they melted and mouldered away
in a dust of blue rain? Who saw the dance of the dead clouds
when the sunlight left them last night, and the west wind blew
them before it like withered leaves?'

John Ruskin (1819–1900)

Ruskin's challenge is about being able to see things more widely.
This is not the language of the television weatherman, who seeks

to impart information derived from scientific measurement. Ruskin wants you to respond to what you observe. He is able to find the words to describe how it was for him.

INTRODUCTION

It is invaluable to go and see, and experience for ourselves, locations that have the power to inspire, to take us out of ourselves and to provide time and space for reflection.

Visits offer:

- a real sense of *time out*
- opportunities to experience the *effects of environment*, landscape and architecture
- a chance to step out of habitual ways of thinking, and to see things from a *different perspective*
- an opportunity to consider the relationship of *form and function*
- a chance to *apply* of all this in medical work, in creating good personal and professional environments.

There is a special quality about a group of professionals on a course who have been given a legitimate freedom of space and time. Doing something different and stimulating and getting outside – a physical shift from the smaller, confined space and rules of the workplace to larger, open spaces – releases energy. The freedom liberates feelings and thoughts that may have been overly confined, and provides a milieu for personal reflection .The opened spaces of the mind are then available for new ideas and for gaining insights and perceptions.

We find that group members enjoy going out on a visit, and that they return with a sense of well-being, relaxed but animated. It is a good lesson.

It is important to understand the effect of our surroundings, so that we can create good environments for medical work, where structure and design are relevant to function and there is comfort (both physically and psychologically) for staff and patients in their relationships with each other and when doing the work. Patients using healthcare buildings can be puzzled by what is going on and where. Buildings need clear visual and spatial markers which can help people and thus reduce fear and uncertainty which often accompanies visits to surgeries and hospitals. Clinical efficiency needs to be balanced with comfort. The environment needs to be welcoming, comfortable and restorative in its own right. For example, the way in which colour and shape are used is significant.

The response to the stories (narratives) that accompany buildings, objects and landscapes – recording their history, what their purposes and functions were and how this was interpreted – can give a wider perspective to human behaviour and how people are in their own spaces.

We suggest visiting places of beauty, great architecture and designed, open spaces that enhance nature, in order to achieve these aims

In order to *illustrate* this, we shall now go from place to place, to find spaces to respond to that have promoted these concepts and made them work. We shall also look at art works that have been placed in, or are part of, environments and what this can engender.

A PLACE OF BEAUTY
FOUNTAINS ABBEY, NORTH YORKSHIRE

'One of the most remarkable places in Europe and a World Heritage Site, comprising the spectacular ruin of a twelfth-century Cistercian Abbey and monastic watermill, an Elizabethan mansion, and one of the best surviving examples of a Georgian water garden. Elegant ornamental lakes ,canals ,temples and cascades provide a succession of dramatic vistas.'

The National Trust Handbook

In 1132, 13 monks sought a place to create their home and workplace and practice their beliefs, where they could survive in a community and be self-sufficient. Four hundred years later, the abbey was closed through the policy of Henry VIII. In the eighteenth century, John Aislabie came across the wild, wooded valley with its abbey ruins. He in turn wished to create a special place to fulfil his beliefs and needs, in this case in beauty in nature, and harness this with architecture.

> **The group task**
> To have time to walk at leisure, alone or with others in the group, through the site and, knowing the history, reflect about the buildings and landscape, what you see, hear and feel. The group then comes together for discussion.

What can happen

Group members become absorbed by the location. They comment on the impact of both the landscape and the architecture, picking out form, symmetry, materials, and the effect of light and space as

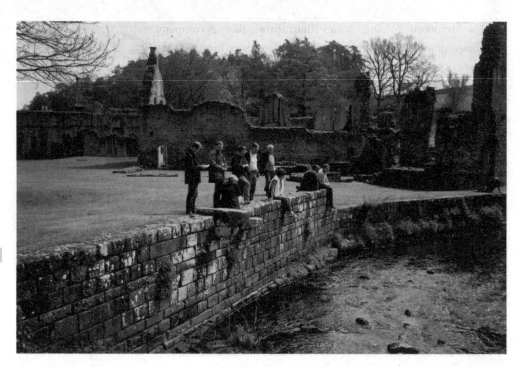

Figure 7.2 A Group at Fountains Abbey

important. They recognise their own sense of well-being, feeling relaxed, their minds stimulated by and engaged with what is around them. They enter imaginatively into the lives of those before them.

'Sitting in the part of the ruins that had been the Infirmary, we started talking about the experience of illness, what it must have been like then, and about how it can still be difficult today. The place affected us.'

SOME LOCATIONS WITH ART INSTALLATIONS/ EXHIBITIONS

A space other than an art gallery can be deliberately used to place and display created works of art.

The environment may complement the nature of the art, give it space and make it easier to view. There may be a theme intended by the artist which links with the function of the building, or which relates to the type of landscape. Art and place together can engender responses. These can extend thinking about links, the significance of form, the artist's creativity and *their* response to the world, adding to what is there and perhaps giving more for us to consider.

Ripon Cathedral

Cathedrals are huge and inspiring spaces, built in a way that promotes intensity of feeling. This magnificent, ancient building was on this occasion also giving space to an art installation entitled *Resurrection* by Anthony Green (Figure 7.3).

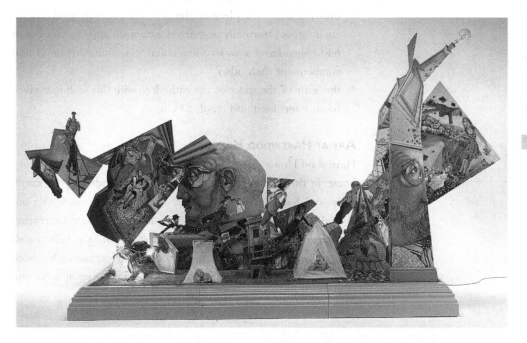

Figure 7.3 *Resurrection* (1996–9), by Anthony Green

This 20-foot-long pictorial sculpture forms a narrative of the artist's life – his representation of his family, relationships and significant events.

A visually exciting work, it gives an insight into the power of recorded memory and how created images of these memories can tell you about the emotions that were experienced. The work is a family album of social history, illness and disease, and the conflicts and joys of relationships. It could have been a version of a family doctor's case records kept over many years and then brought to life – the contexts given understanding and meaning to all aspects of a person's life.

Narrative has always had a place and significance in cathedrals, more usually visually, relayed by the stories unfolded on stain glass windows, and by wood and stone carvings. This huge, carnival-float-like structure, situated in the special space of the building, was an addition to the human story in an arresting and compelling way, its modern images adding to those already placed to record in previous times.

At this visit, the group's responses included:

1 interest and excitement at the artist's imagination and ability to represent social history in this way
2 a resultant curiosity to know what it was all about and what story each part of the sculpture was telling
3 thinking about the place of the art work in a cathedral (not an environment normally associated with this), and the fact that it had engendered a wider view about how things relate to and complement each other
4 the sense of the space of the cathedral, with this sculpture given room – included and cradled by it.

ART AT HAREWOOD HOUSE

Harewood House was built in the grand style of the great country house in the eighteenth century and is surrounded by parkland, lakes and formal gardens (Figure 7.4). Thus in this setting are several man-made environments, the formal geometric terracing and gardens leading the eye to the open spaces of lake, hills, woods created from the original natural topography. Here nature has been adjusted so that we can see the most pleasing shapes of trees and water, for our aesthetic enjoyment.

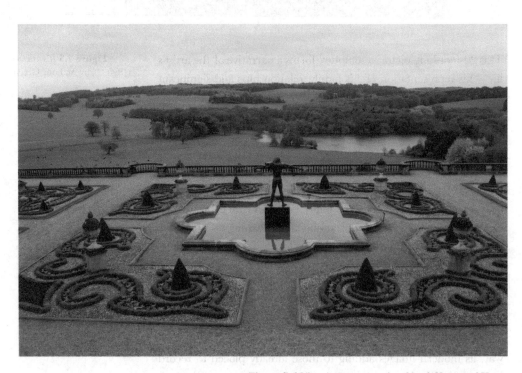

Figure 7.4 Victorian terrace and parkland, Harewood House

There is an art-exhibition space, housed on the ground floor of the main house, for changing exhibitions, which opens out onto the garden terraces.

We saw *Out of place* here, an exhibition by contemporary international artists of work created to express ideas of place and location, and the need, and indeed the urge, of humans to connect with the world. In doing this they showed that there are many different definitions, rather than fixed meanings of things, encouraging viewers to look enquiringly, to question assumptions and to comprehend in a wider way.

Examples from some of the exhibits

1 A video installation showed a workman painting and stencilling a *STOP* sign at a road junction. The action had been slowed down, the photography picking out and emphasising the workman's balance, and his hands and feet. It had become a beautiful synchronised ballet of colour and movement, showing the grace and skill of an ordinary act. The activity had been re-interpreted, seen differently and given a significance of its own, rather than a fixed mechanistic meaning, and encouraged the viewer to think imaginatively.

2 The second example depicted a bleak, city open street, with snow and sleet falling. The fixed camera position showed the arrival of people at a bus stop, the bus eventually arriving, and a person still there as the bus drove away, who then wandered off, head down, along the street. This emphasised the narrative that can come with spaces – how recorded factual happenings, also become fictional, as stories or ideas created from what we see. Who was the solitary figure? Why didn't they get on the bus? Were they meeting someone who didn't arrive? Space is made significant by what happens in it.

3 This example was a series of images showing a room with a balcony in an apartment block. The same room was repeated many times, from the same viewpoint, but in each separate picture the room was filled with different possessions and had a different layout, and each time it created a different atmosphere or feeling.

The images in this exhibit contrasted enormously with the view on leaving the exhibition, of Capability Brown's great design for nature in the landscape stretching ahead. Stepping in and out of frames in this way, the images that we see bump into each other and generate new ideas and new perspectives, which is what much of the work described in this book is aiming to do. Sometimes to see the picture, you *have* to step outside the frame.

What we hoped to achieve

• *Recognising comfort zones*

For some it was easier to enjoy the beautiful, familiar and accepted pattern of landscaped nature, seen on emerging from the exhibition room, than to meet the demand by the artists to comprehend modern environments and objects from a different view. To remain always in an area which is familiar can be a limit to development. Medical work involves acquiring new techniques and understanding many views and attitudes.

Overcoming fear of the unknown and knowing how to manage challenging situations is important otherwise, there is a denial of and failure to follow through significant events, because either we can't face it or we don't know what to do. Recognising responses, and being helped to find ways of change in order to cope, can be invaluable.

• *Making connections*

Recognising the importance and significance of the arrangement and content of personal environments, as shown in some of the exhibits, can directly relate to the experience of healthcare practitioners when visiting patients in their own homes. There is a need to comprehend, understand and accept, to be interested in how people live, and to be free of prejudice and assumptions which can cause difficulties in communication. The way people order their lives tells us a lot about them.

YORKSHIRE SCULPTURE PARK

Figure 7.5 *Reclining Figure, Arch Leg* (1969–70), by Henry Moore

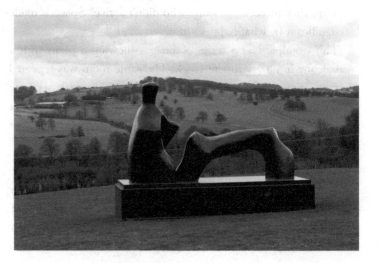

'Sculpture is an art of the open air. Daylight, sunlight is necessary to it. I would rather have a piece of my sculpture put in a landscape, almost any landscape, than on or in, the most beautiful building I know.'

Henry Moore

There are 500 acres of landscape – rolling eighteenth-century woodland, lakes and terraces – at Bretton Park to provide a glorious environment for some of the best examples of contemporary sculpture. A 2-hour walk leads through this landscape, providing views of magnificent shapes and groupings of trees, patterns of light on water, and the combination of the sky and the undulating hills. The forms and textures of the sculptures among this provide a complementary extension of the landscape's visual impact . The space and light of the setting enable an appreciation of the three-dimensional shapes. You can touch the sculptures and place yourself next to their size and presence, you can begin to feel the artists' creativity and understand the translation of their ideas into these forms.

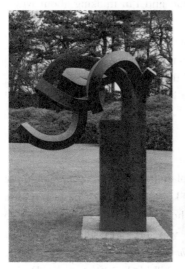 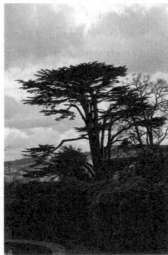

Figure 7.6 *Peine del Viento XVII* (1990), by Eduardo Chillida

Figure 7.7 Trees at Yorkshire Sculpture Park

A walk in the sculpture park
Consider   What do you see?   What do you feel?
Things to reflect about as you walk:

- the sculpture's relationship with the environment
- the environment in its own right
- light and space
- form and function
- what the sculptures are about for you – is meaning important?

Each member of the group had a map showing the walk and sculpture placements. They elected to be independent and not go as a guided tour, but elected for self-discovery, singly or in twos or threes. At the end of the trip we talked about it together.

What did they say?
- 'It was very good together with some of the others, talking about what we seeing and discovering what their ideas and views were. I learnt a lot.'
- 'I find sculpture quite difficult, and I'm thinking about why I feel like that.'
- 'It was very relaxing, I've come back feeling very open to things.'
- 'The greatest work of all was the landscape.'
- 'When I climbed into one of the sculptures I realised the metaphor of my own involvement in getting at the inside of things.'

DESIGN

Design is about working out, planning and inventing something that has an intended function. The function may be in response to a perceived need (e.g. the hospital as a specialised place to treat illness), or it may be a way of expressing an idea, an emotion (e.g. the sculpture *The Angel of the North* by Anthony Gormley, arms outstretched on a hillside by a motorway). Design will involve artistry, technology and economics. It reflects the results of social development. Good design will take into account practical usage, as well as embracing cultural, psychological and ecological aspects.

Here is an exercise that involves practising designing an 'environment', applying some of the thoughts and ideas perhaps stimulated by an outside visit.

DESIGN YOUR OWN CONSULTING ROOM

This is a group exercise in which people first work in subgroups of three or four individuals.

Materials needed in advance include model rooms and furniture – chairs, desks, examination couches, doors, computers and keyboards, windows, and a selection of micro paintings, as in a doll's house. Old cardboard boxes that have a side cut out and are then painted and papered can be the rooms. The furniture can be made, using matchboxes, wooden tongue depressors and balsa wood.

Each small group is given one of the rooms and the pieces of furniture.

Each group chooses its paintings from a common collection, which should range from Old Masters through to the abstract (perhaps downloaded from the Internet). Also provide blank frames for groups to add anything else they want.

> Using the room and furniture, etc. they have been given, each subgroup should design the room as they would like it, and then present this to the rest of the group, explaining the reasons for their design.

What happens

1 Learners quickly get very absorbed in this exercise and are instantly animated by it. It draws in even the most reticent group member.

2 When placing furniture, etc., group members focus on the needs of the patients and staff using the room. For example, they start thinking how users will want to sit in the consultation so that they can see each other without a computer screen being in the way.

3 Group members think about windows – giving light appropriately, the view (and its content) enhancing or distracting – and they debate the effect of closed blinds, etc. This leads to further discussion about how it feels in consultations, both for patients and professionals, if the space seems too enclosed and oppressive.

4 Safety issues are addressed. Should a patient become aggressive, is the desk in a position where the professional is not going to be hemmed in? This discussion will be a vehicle for releasing any concerns about dealing with aggression.

5 The choice of paintings will enable a debate about their function (e.g. something that is seen as restful and soothing, something containing plenty of activity and colour to talk about with children). Are the pictures for the benefit of the room holder – something they like, and something that relates to their own leisure interest?

6 The blank picture frames act as a focus for discussing personal material(e.g. family photographs, certificates showing qualifications). This can continue into extended group work about the nature of the patient/professional relationship and how much identifying material we want revealed, and its significance in the relationship.

7 There is recognition of the need to have workplaces that are not just functional, but also personally satisfying, so that there is no discomfort of the mind or body to distract from doing a good job.

Figure 7.8 *We keep buying things 'that'll look better', and it just doesn't.* From *Signs of the Times* (1992), by Martin Parr

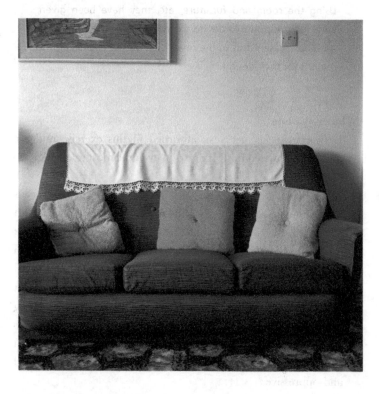

In conclusion

The experience of environment, appreciating design and its significance, can be applied to working in medical practice. Practical activity gives learners opportunities to examine their imaginative responses, attitudes and knowledge as things happen. Future action and thinking in other environments can benefit from this experience.

8 TAKE ONE

TEACHING WITH FILM

Films (movies) embrace many of the art forms that we have already discussed, such as image, narrative, drama, music and, of course, location. Many students find that film is the most accessible arts medium because of its familiar format (most people have experience of watching films either on TV or at the cinema), and so many tutors new to using arts resources may find it the easiest to use.

Here is a *detailed work through* of the process of using film as an arts resource in teaching. The example shows the use of a *film extract*.

1 SETTING THE AIM

In this example the **educational aim** is *looking at communication skills with adolescents* – the *intention* of this session is to illustrate how young people may behave and respond in a life crisis situation, to enable the learner to observe this response and understand the best course of action, to be aware of their own feelings and emotions, and then to practise communicating effectively as a result.

2 FINDING AND SELECTING THE RESOURCE

Select something that catches the drama of a moment, that tells a story, that pares down, refines and simplifies what needs to be absorbed, that creates the appearance of reality, and that will be accepted as 'true' while we watch. Where we can react with the characters, feel their distress, anger and joy at what is happening, perhaps wanting them to do things differently as we perceive different solutions. The compelling immediacy of a film can displace other things occupying the mind – it is an alternative activity, a change from routine work, and so perhaps allows space for emotions to be expressed which are otherwise held in check.

CHOSEN RESOURCE

We have selected a 10–15 minute extract, from Jane Campion's film *An Angel at my Table*. This film traces the life of the writer Janet Frame in New Zealand, from childhood, through an episode of intense psychological breakdown as a young woman, and then on to success. In the episode chosen, she is in her teens and living with her family. Her sister drowns in a swimming accident when Janet is not present, having declined to go swimming with her as she preferred to do something else. The news of the tragedy is given to the mother by a doctor, who is insensitive and also ignores Janet. Her subsequent grieving is alone, and her own plight in bereavement appears not to have been acknowledged by anyone.

3 DESIGNING THE EXERCISE

A small group will watch the extract, and then have a facilitated discussion about it.

PRACTICAL POINT

Always *check* the video/DVD player and screen before your teaching session starts, making sure it is working and that you know how to use it.

BEFORE SHOWING THE EXTRACT

Before showing the film extract, give a brief 'the story so far ...' introduction. Prepare this beforehand so that you are fluent and can communicate the essential information to make the *context* of the extract comprehensible – that is, who the characters are and what the location is, but without revealing what you want the learners to perceive for themselves.

4 ACHIEVING ENGAGEMENT

You are using the film extract to access feelings, perceptions and ideas that you want the group to provide.

Be clear in your own mind about your aim in using the extract, but remember that you want the group to do the work. So in the *guidance to learners* on how they watch the extract, it is better to say:

> *'Please take note of what you see, hear and feel when the doctor arrives at the family home',*

not

> *'Look how insensitive the doctor's approach is, and how upset the girl appears to be.'*

When the extract finishes there is usually total silence as the learners are still absorbed with the film. Don't worry – just wait a bit for everyone to get back to the present.

5 FACILITATING RESPONSES

Request *first thoughts* from the group.

EXAMPLES

'I didn't think much of how that doctor broke bad news.'
'She was a bit of a wimp, wasn't she? I mean, it wasn't her fault her sister died, you'd think she'd just get on with it.'
'Oh, I found it very moving. I don't what to say.'

Elicit what has prompted these replies.

'You say you were unimpressed by the doctor. Can you describe what you saw, and what you perceived the girl's response was, and how this was portrayed by the film maker? Comments from anyone else about this?'

Encourage reflection about emotions and feelings expressed.

'I'm wondering what it was in the film that made you feel so strongly about what you just said?'

Look at application of gained knowledge/insights, and relate to previous experience.

'I had a patient who drowned – it's only just occurred to me that I never got a chance to talk to her brother.'
'Yes, I wonder now if the brother were here, what you would like to say to him, what phrases would you use?'

Summarise learning.

'You've been able to see and feel what can happen to this adolescent girl as she experiences a sudden death in her family. We've looked at some of the ways you might be able to talk to her, and understand her needs. Next time you are breaking bad news, helping a bereaved young person, some of this may be of use.'

6 FEEDBACK

Getting feedback will give some indication of whether your aims have been met, whether the resource and exercise were appropriate, and whether your teaching style was clear, acceptable and effective.

What you hope will have happened by the end of the session and confirmed in feedback is that:

- events and patterns in human behaviour have been recognised (e.g. in this example, relating to the loss of a family member)
- group members have gained insights from each other about their different experiences in watching the same film extract
- negative responses such as impatience have given way to understanding
- disturbing emotions have been shared, carried and managed
- opportunities to rehearse and to consider the effect of words and phrases in communication have been used
- further learning needs have been expressed – for example, the need for a session on how to break bad news
- group members enjoyed working in a different way, and that they found watching the film a stimulating experience, and understood what the session had been about.

Here are some **more examples** of the possibilities for using film in teaching for you to think about. How would you do it?

- As part of a **travel medicine** workshop.
  Aim – to focus on the psychological trauma that can be associated with illness while travelling, and enable medical personnel to understand the experience of unexpected, life threatening events, how people may behave and react, and what their needs will be.
  Suggestion: The Sheltering Sky *by Bernado Bertolucci, showing a death in the desert.*
- For **communication skills** training.
  Aim – to focus on the complexity of relationships, particularly in families, and on how to understand what may be going on (which may be disguised as a health problem).
  Suggestion: Secrets and Lies *by Mike Leigh, showing the twenty-first birthday party.*
- As part of a workshop on **mental health in the elderly**.
  Aim – to focus on patients' insights, dilemmas and behaviour in progressive diseases.
  Suggestion: Iris, *Judi Dench's portrayal of Iris Murdoch's life with Alzheimer's disease.*
- As part of a workshop on **ethics**.
  Aim – to illustrate the emotions of dilemma when a moral problem may be involved.
  Suggestion: Onegin, *with Ralph Fiennes. The duel episode and what leads up to it.*

9 THE DRAMA OF EVERYDAY LIFE

David Powley

The work discussed in this chapter offers another opportunity for healthcare practitioners to express themselves creatively, by involving them directly as active participants in drama, as actors, directors and audience.

As in all of the previous chapters, the work is designed to engage learners with their personal experience of life. It does this in the first half by starting from that experience and giving dramatic shape to it. Then it moves on to starting with the given shape of existing drama texts and working back into personal experience.

The bulk of what follows focuses on working with a group, but it could be adapted to working with individuals. And once again the structures are not rigid. They may be varied according to need or desired outcome or in response to what happens during the work.

Two things are important in this work:

1 the *content of the drama* (i.e. the stories themselves, personal or otherwise)
2 what is going on in *the process of working with drama* as a medium.

The content is deeply influenced by the process of giving our experience dramatic form, much as it would be when working within any other art form. That process is like a journey in which we discover bit by bit more about the nature of that experience and our relationship to it. 'Drama' offers us as participants, however 'unskilled' in the craft we may think we are, surprisingly easy and immediate access to our creativity, once we have taken the first leap.

The 'process of working' involves both the way we respond to the experience itself, in which we develop a dramatic 'eye' for things, and the honing of dramatic skills. The latter includes, for example, developing our awareness of how we use the body and voice, and the space we 'act' in.

This chapter goes into some detail about this 'process', even with what may seem, on the face of it very simple acts, partly to demonstrate that more is going on than we may think, partly to lay down some principles of action for the work as a whole, and partly because the process itself encourages the development of useful and creative ways of seeing and responding to experience in our everyday lives, that may be otherwise unrecognised or underused or even suppressed.

What distinguishes drama from the rest of the arts? In a word – *action*. Through action, the *whole person* is engaged – physically, mentally and emotionally – responding to and influencing other people and things and the space that contains us.

This can only happen if the people concerned *allow* themselves to be thus engaged. Involving oneself in action, especially in a group, with so many pairs of eyes as witness, can feel exposed and embarrassing. Resistance can be high. So we need to *ease* ourselves into engagement.

There are a number of ways of doing this. For example, we can:

- provide a clear and safe framework to what we do
- proceed in simple incremental steps
- encourage a relaxed attitude and atmosphere in which the crippling notion of 'failure' can take a back seat and playing can be fun
- warm ourselves up.

WORKING FROM PERSONAL EXPERIENCE
GETTING STARTED

1 The room
The room needs to be big enough for the number of people you (the workshop facilitator) are working with to move around freely and to work in smaller groups, each with enough territory to protect them from the others. The work in small groups could benefit from a few break-out rooms, as a refuge from noise.

Although the room may be big enough, it is unlikely to be empty. Before people arrive, clear the room of all excess furniture and equipment and make sure there is a clear, out-of-the-way place for people to deposit things they bring with them. Ideally, you should be left with an empty room, except for enough chairs to seat the group, arranged in a circle in the middle.

This is not simply about maximising the space available. In so far as it contrasts with functional spaces the participants are used to, such as seminar rooms with chairs in rows facing a screen, the nearly empty room also makes a statement and prompts a question about what may happen here. It may thus be a little unsettling, which is good (in small doses) for shaking creativity free. It also gives a clear opportunity to create other spaces within it, like writing on a blank page, and that in turn is about transformation, which is an essential of what we shall be doing in this room through drama.

However, the circle of chairs in the centre gives the reassurance of the familiar, or at least of a clear place to go to, whether we like sitting in circles or not. It is a clear structure.

A good deal of what we'll do in this space is about being clear. For example, if we set a scene for a drama we have created, the clarity with which the 'set' is defined will affect the clarity of how we play it and of how our audience receives it. The clearer we are, the more we can both discover and reveal through our drama. And revelation is another essential of drama.

Whether you clear the room yourself or get the group to help you depends on how dramatic you want to be. Entering a ready-prepared 'set' raises expectations and questions, which can be a good thing. On the other hand, if members of the group do the clearing with you, people have something practical to do, which is comforting, and they begin working together physically. Most importantly, it involves everyone in a transformation, the first of many to come, and of the space itself. And they begin to take possession of it.

2 Sitting in the circle

When everybody has sat down, talk just enough to give a basic idea of what the work will be about; but also enough for anyone, whether they are familiar or not with active drama work, to acknowledge what they feel about it in anticipation. It is normal to find a mixture of anxiety, curiosity and excitement. A matter-of-fact admission and acceptance of it (and sharing it with fellow participants) relaxes people a little. It also sets the tone – it's all right to feel and say these things, because they *are* quite normal and human. Then you can get on with the action. However, there is one thing commonly encountered at this stage: 'But I can't act!'

This is relevant to healthcare workers:

- in the organisation of their work spaces and in enabling their patients to feel comfortable in them (see 'Design' in Chapter 7, 'Out on location')

- because how they think about their physical space is a mirror of how they think about their work in general and their relationship with patients. In fact, all that follows in this chapter is an active metaphor, and therefore exploration and practice, for how they work and are as people.

The first leap! The problem is that most people think of 'acting' only as a specialist professional activity and as 'Acting' with a capital 'A'. The fact is that 'acting' with a small 'a' is what we do all the time in our everyday lives. Engaging with experience through a dramatic framework is what we do automatically in order to survive. It is one of the things that make us human.

Among the essentials of drama are the twin notions of 'what if' and 'as if'. 'What if the world I am about to enter is ... "this" ... "that" ... or the "other"?'. 'If it is "this", then maybe I need to behave in a "this" way.' And so we model our behaviour in a way we judge to be appropriate in a 'this' context and we behave 'as if' our judgement were true. Then we find out if we're right. If we are, we stride forward with confidence in our 'this' world. If not, then we need to adjust – which we may find hard to do.

Equally, we often reflect on past action, saying, 'what if (or if only) I had behaved differently'. We even replay the scenes, sometimes repeatedly, partially in the head but often also, when we think no one is looking, with little movements and bits of speech. Thus we learn, we hope, a little bit about doing better next time.

We are forever devising new scenarios to test out and adapt to. And we are forever prone to settling so comfortably into certain of them that it comes as a shock when we have to conjure up another one to meet changing circumstances, or perhaps when we feel ourselves getting stuck in ruts too deeply cut and want badly enough to climb out.

We are engaged in this dialectic all the time. Most of the time, we are unaware of it. Just as we don't normally think about the mechanics of walking or talking, because we are so used to doing it, so we don't think about our everyday 'acting' – until circumstances change in a big way (e.g. going for an interview for a new job). Then we do become conscious of 'what-iffing', and of rehearsing – in front of a mirror, even. We may not think of it as an elemental form of 'drama', but it is.

The richness of our lives depends a great deal on how adept we are at 'playing' appropriately a range of 'roles', which is what adapting our behaviour in essence amounts to: finding the 'role' (or a set of attributes or characteristics) within us, with which to shape most effectively our response to others and the circumstances we find ourselves in. Our sense of who we are develops from our 'what-if/as-if' forays and how we seek to extend or limit them . Ultimately, perhaps, our sense of fulfilment depends on finding and living through the 'roles' and 'scenarios' that are best suited to us.

The better we are at the 'art' of 'drama', the better we are at the 'art' of living and the better chance we have of fulfilment.

So, we can all 'act' – or, if we can't, then we're in real trouble.

3 The action starts

Now comes that awkward moment of leaving the safety of our chairs. What follows is a series of small doses of action for you to administer, increasing at each stage in dramatic strength.

(i) Crossing the circle

The instructions are written as a guide for what the facilitator tells the group. Make up your own variations and do as many as seems appropriate.

- Make and hold eye contact with someone else in the circle (the facilitator should join in with this).
- As soon as contact is established (it has to be mutually recognised) get up, cross the circle and sit in the other person's chair.
- Now find another person's eyes. When contact is made, get up, cross circle and sit down. Speed it up. Another person. Find the eyes more quickly. Make contact with as many people as possible. Cross the circle and sit down.
- Now, as you cross, stop briefly in front of each other to say your name (if people don't know each other) or 'hallo'. Encourage them to make the stop very brief but very precise. So, make contact first, then get up, etc.
- Maybe add observing what the other person is wearing and simply naming one thing (e.g. 'blue shirt').
- Do again but with physical contact. For example, greet each other in different ways, from shaking hands to touching palms to something silly, like a quick pat-a-cake. All with words/ sounds.
- Now be more elaborate. Imagine you are all very stately elegant dancers at a ball. Briefly dance stylishly with the other – but your partner's chair pulls you to it before you can become too carried away. Again add words/sound.
- Contrast this by crossing in as grotesque a manner as possible. Be big, brutish and noisy, sniffing suspiciously and growling at your partner as you circle each other and pass on to the allotted chair.

If you have no experience of doing this sort of thing and are a little reticent by nature, these exercises may strike you as so daft that you couldn't imagine yourself doing them. This is partly

So for healthcare workers the relevance of 'acting' and experiencing that process through the drama is clear.

- They are in everyday life 'acting' very specific roles, often in an unnecessarily restricted manner. How can they be broadened while retaining their essential characteristics?

- They can gain an inner understanding of patient behaviour and how they act out the 'dramas' which are their lives.

the effect of translating action into the reduced outlines of cold print. But also the exercises really are, in fact, on one level, 'daft' in that they do invite us to play like children and to be what we might normally class as 'silly'. They encourage us to loosen up.

But they are also very tightly structured, so that each stage in their development is in itself simple. Here you can see the whole package in one go, whereas in practice participants wouldn't know what was coming next. All they know is that something is going to happen, which may provoke a little anxiety, but then the ease of doing no more than crossing the circle to another's chair comes as a bit of a relief.

The circle produces a small and contained space in which each journey across it – each exposure – is brief and so relatively unthreatening. Most of the rules remain the same – make eye contact, stand, cross over and sit down. Repetition quickly establishes the skill required to do this snappily, without thinking about it, and that leaves people free to become increasingly inventive and extravagant with the one variable – the way they relate to each other as they cross.

Add to this pace and momentum. Keeping it going, allowing only brief rests as the next ingredient is introduced or a bit of technique is sharpened (e.g. the precision of stopping and starting, greeting, parting, etc.) generates energy rather than letting it seep away. Then, of course, there is the participants' engagement with it. The laughter that is generated even with the first couple of crossings and the spontaneous applause often prompted by this or that couple doing something particularly inventive, produce their own momentum.

As the exercise progresses, the invitations become bigger and more extravagant and, through contrasting extremes, briefly extends everyone physically, vocally and emotionally. The circle acts as a crucible in which spontaneous play bursts briefly into life, but also in which participants begin to ingest, through practice, a small sense of dramatic structure and technical discipline, and to awaken the body to the possibilities of movement and voice; all of which will be built on as you progress further.

Finally, it is up to the facilitator to catch the rhythm and tone of the group, to time the addition of ingredients and tightening of technique, without inhibiting invention by over-direction. All that is probably best done from within, as a fellow participant.

(ii) Breaking the circle

- Make something of the transition, even if only to say, 'So, we've been in this cosy little circle for a bit. Now we'll break out of it.' Let the thought settle. Stand up. Each person takes their own chair to stack well out of the way. Make sure that this is done such that the space is as free of them as possible. Even in this, pay attention to detail.
- Now make two lines, facing each other, of equal numbers, facing into the room (the leader can join in). 'Now we're ready for the "no flies" game.'
- One line moves first, walking towards the other line as a group, chanting at them the following:

> 'there ain't no flies on us, there ain't no flies on us,
> there may be flies on some of you guys
> but there ain't no flies on us!'

The first line stops just before it reaches the other and runs back to the wall it's just come from. It turns and faces the other line as it does the same and runs back. Having established the mechanics, now play with it. It's a 'naughty children's' game, a taunting game, a challenging ritual between one gang and another. Play it as large as possible, and let yourselves go with it. Act as a group, all picking up on the kind of movement and tone at any one foray.

- Change the speed and the tone. For example, try doing it seductively. Individuals can initiate other ways of advancing on the opposite gang, the rest of the gang picking up on their lead.
- End it by both groups moving towards each other and stopping a metre apart, but putting a lot of energy into the nose-thumbing challenge. 'OK. Relax.'

The little ritual at the beginning with the chairs is not in itself important, but it does build on the idea that transitions are of special importance and are worth marking both in drama and in life; that any moment can be given dramatic form and thus be heightened; and that paying attention to the way we define our space is important.

4 Sculptures

- Find a partner, and together move to a space in the room as far away from everyone else as possible (if there is an odd number in the group, the facilitator can join in). Use the whole room. Just stand quietly for a moment, shut your eyes

Relevance of crossing the circle and breaking the circle to healthcare workers

- Being able to relax and play is not just about preparing for playing with drama, it is about letting loose creativity, an energy that flows from the 'child' in everyone, and which can be healthily active in their healthcare work.

- Working with clear structures and forms that enable in themselves and in their patients a creative spontaneity that may lead to insights beyond the obvious, thus making the consultation more fulfilling.

and think of what has happened so far today, from getting up to being here (or some other recent time, no more than a day long). Flip through the files in your mind to view the various minor incidents and scenes that have made up your day. With each minor (or major) event you will have *felt* something (e.g. amusement, pleasure, joy, anxiety, irritation, anger), not necessarily epic in proportion, but at least feelings that stand out a bit from the rest. Settle on one of these. Indicate when you have found one. As long as one person per pair has one, you can start. Getting on with the task gives time for memories to work.

- One of you will be a sculptor and the other a large lump of clay, ready to be turned into a work of art. Choose who will be which of these. You will swap over later. The task is for the sculptors to sculpt their clay into a statue that expresses the feeling remembered in the incident they have just chosen. It externalises and physically enlarges what may have been largely an internal event, so make the finished sculpture as physically exaggerated as possible.

- Stick to the following rules of the game. Don't tell your clay anything through speech. You have two methods open to you to achieve the shape you wish for (within the physical limits of your bit of clay!). One is to shape them by physically altering the position and posture of their bodies – hands on sculpting! The other, useful when trying to achieve the quality and intensity of expression, is to demonstrate these things yourself, for your sculpture to copy – but purely through bodily expression, not speech.

- Work quickly and intuitively. Allow about 5 minutes. Stop the action when it looks as though most have finished.

- The sculptures should hold their positions for their creators to inspect, then relax out of them, then take them up again. Can you remember exactly how you were shaped? Sculptors should refine their work, and sculptures hold positions. All of the sculptors should have a quick look at other people's work, an exhibition of statues. Note and admire the range, then return to your own sculpture.

- Now the sculptures do the following.

  1 First, let the physicality of your sculpted body – its position, intensity and quality – give you a sense of the feelings giving rise to them in yourself, and let the feelings grow.

2 Let both the physical shape you have been given and the feelings aroused begin to translate into movement on the spot.

3 Then let an appropriate sound emerge, and increase both movement and sound.

4 Next let the movement take you across space

5 Then let the sound translate into a few words and phrases that seem to express the feelings.

6 Let whatever suggests itself to you come out. Never mind whether you know what the circumstances were in reality for your creator. You have a life of your own now.

7 All this should take only a minute or two.

• Now stop and relax. Have a brief debrief with your partner – but in the following order.

1 The sculptures check whether what they did caught something of what their sculptor's feelings were – but sculptors don't at this stage explain or tell the story of the event. Let the sculptures say what they felt it was all about.

2 Let the sculptors give feedback.

• Then swap over and start again.
• When the whole process is complete for the second time, give the pairs 2 or 3 minutes to talk to each other about the experience of doing this exercise, making a note of things they learned or found interesting.
• Give brief feedback (e.g. one observation from each pair) to the whole group.

Here the whole space is being used, but at the same time care is taken to find and define pair-spaces within it. It drip-feeds a sense of boundaries – physical frames that keep the work clear – and different ways of being separate and together in the same space. This continues to happen throughout these exercises, for space, and how we define and move in it, is one of the principal materials of dramatic expression, just as the framed space of a canvas is for the painter.

The exercise has now become more sharply focused and lasts for longer. The stages through which it passes encourage clarity, attention to detail and quality, without being too demanding, with attention directed in particular to quality of feelings and the body through which they are to be expressed. Both as sculptors and as the clay we become more acutely aware not just of our partner's body, but also of our own, and of just what our own bodies do to express feelings. And then we do a little bit of body memory training in letting the shape go and bringing it back.

Invariably people are surprised by how accurately their sculpture partners play back their feelings and thoughts (and even recognise the situation itself) when they are brought to life. And even if the words or the scenarios that suggest themselves to the sculptures seem on the surface to derive from quite different events to those specifically experienced by the sculptors, a little discussion soon reveals that they most often share the same underlying pattern of experience and the same basic feelings.

The relief of being allowed back into speech at the end imparts enormous energy to group members' feedback to each other, in which the stories of these moments of feeling can be told more fully.

What is happening in this exercise brings us back to our ability to imagine scenarios and our roles within them. This ability has another dimension to it that is essential both to the drama process and to our sense of self. We can also imagine what it is like to be other people, or creatures, or even things – animate and inanimate.

From ancient times this ability was given detailed and refined form in, for example, hunting rituals, which were in effect rehearsals, when humans took on the characteristics of the animals that they were about to hunt, sometimes even dressing up as them, partly so they would be better at predicting the animals' behaviour. They took it very seriously because success in the hunt really mattered.

And this ability still really matters to us. Certainly, it still enables us to 'know' and perhaps outwit our prey or our enemy. Indeed, the rehearsal in front of the mirror for an interview has much in common with what the hunter does. The dressing up, the adaptations of speech, and the physical bearing and movement are not simply dreamt up, but derive from observation of the types of people we think we have to impress and the types of people we think have been successful applicants in the past; all of which is informed by received wisdom from our particular tribe about the form these events should take – the rules of the game.

However, this kind of empathic knowing also acts as a conduit for compassion, friendship and love, and sharing what is common to us all. This in turn may nurture into growth something in us that hitherto had lain dormant, thus expanding our sense of our selves and our potential 'roles', which we may then rehearse in the world at large. Or we may be more likely to try out what we see or feel others do, thus perhaps finding another 'role' that fits.

5 Listening to the stories

Version (i)

- Stay in pairs, with the same partner. (Here it is perhaps better for the facilitator to step out of the action and for the bereft partner to join another pair to make a three.) Sit opposite each other so you can easily hear what you say to each other. One of you will be the teller and the other the listener. Choose who will be which.
- Now the teller has just 4 minutes (the facilitator should time the group of three separately so that they each have about 3 minutes) to tell the listener(s) everything about the day so far, from getting up to sitting here. *The listener must just listen, with no verbal interruption, no questions or comment.* Even if there is a silence because the teller has apparently run out of things to tell, listeners should resist the temptation to jump to the rescue. Just let the silence be, and let the teller think about how to enlarge upon what has already been said and then do it.
- Note that people are in charge of what they choose to tell. They are not expected to tell things that they would prefer to keep to themselves.
- The facilitator should time the 4 minutes and then stop the talk, whether tellers have finished or not, by asking them to bring the part they are in the middle of to a rapid close. Now the listeners should just store what they have heard until later – for the time being everyone will swap roles and the new listener will hear the new teller's story for another 4 minutes.
- Now both members of the pair think about the stories they have heard and how they felt themselves responding to them. Some parts will have caught their attention or interest, or engaged their feeling, more fully than others. Each person should choose one such moment or episode to explore further.
- The first listener now asks the first teller the sort of enabling questions that will help to explore and open up that episode and follow through as they hear the answers. Discover something more about the feelings that were expressed (or not) in the event described. Just take about 3 minutes over this, again timed by the facilitator. Then swap roles again.
- Now everyone should relax from all these rules and have a brief discussion in their pairs of what doing all this was like and what

This exercise is relevant to healthcare workers in its encouragement of our ability to empathise with others – another way of knowing people and ourselves. It stresses the role of the body in that process. We 'listen' with it and to it. It is not just a matter of spotting body language and being able to interpret it. It is a way of sensing what it is like to be other people, so that we may resonate with them and find something of them in ourselves, and of ourselves in them.

they noticed about how they felt while doing it. Each pair should decide on one or two things they found most interesting about it, to feed back to the whole group.

A shorter version of this exercise, though with the same structure, could be as follows.

Version (ii)

- After the sculptures exercise, find a new partner.
- Tell just one episode from the day so far that seemed most strongly felt by you, the teller. Take 2 minutes. It could be the one you used in making the sculpture, or a different one.
- Listeners then ask opening-up questions about that for 2 minutes.
- There is a short debriefing as before.

How fascinating and revealing people's ordinary everyday lives are! That is the reaction most people have, doing this exercise. How much happens. How much we recognise as similar to our own lives. How much our routines also vary ('Really? I must try that?'). How intimate is the glimpse we have into other people's lives, and how revealing these everyday rituals and events are of who we are and how we live. The stories provoke a lot of laughter and shared concern, even if the listeners cannot respond in words.

We shouldn't be so surprised by this as, after all, the fabric of our lives is woven from these everyday stories – what we do every day and how we do it. Yet most of these moments are passed by, usually without a second's thought, and often they are lost altogether, taken for granted, in the rush to get from one minute to the next. Yet how we handle our passage from one small episode to the next is a pretty good indication of our state of health. And so is how much we are able to recall and re-enter these moments.

This listening exercise is a little 'what-if/as-if' drama in its own right. The listeners are taking on a role they may not normally so clearly inhabit, as solely 'the listener'. Participants most often observe that they do have urges to intervene with a question or with examples from their own experience. Some take a little while to settle into a way of listening that feels natural and present, without words. Similarly, some tellers feel a little disorientated by having all the time to themselves to speak in an uninterrupted manner. Some feel the need for more feedback, especially approval, while others are only too happy to be listened to.

Any intervention on the part of the listener will alter what is then said, and is often more about the listeners listening for a chance to tell their own stories. Keeping quiet gives the teller a chance really to think about what they have done, knowing that silences will not otherwise be snatched away from them. How we respond during this 4 minutes (which is longer than it may seem on paper!) can in itself be instructive.

The chance to ask opening-up questions relieves this tension, but it also invites those asking the questions to become more aware of their own responses. It also encourages them to adopt the drama mind-set that asks the basic question 'what is going on?'.

6 Retelling the stories

- Get into groups of four (with a six or a five, if numbers dictate).
- Within the groups each person's chosen story will be told to the rest of the group, whether it was chosen by your partner's interest in it, as in Version 5(i) above, or by you, as in Version 5(ii) above. However, *you will not tell your episode yourself.* The person who originally listened to you will. And those listeners will tell it in a special way – in the first person, as if they were you and it was their story.
- See if you can settle a bit into how your partner sits and moves, and the tone and movement (rather than pitch and accent!) of their voice.
- As each little story is finished, 'as-if' tellers check briefly with the original tellers to establish whether they got it right.
- Now have a brief feedback session on what the exercise felt like.

Many people feel nervous about speaking as if they were their partners. What if they get it wrong? They feel responsible, especially if the story itself involves strong feelings, or they worry what they will seem like if they can't remember it! Meanwhile, if you are the original teller, you may well feel odd, seeing 'yourself' in action, as well as concerned that you are not misrepresented. So for both parties the check at the end of each story is important. It establishes a protocol that in turn helps to establish trust between participants, but it also practises the art of stepping into someone else's shoes and taking on another role – all of which is relevant to the healthcare professional.

7 Seeing the stories in still images
(i) As one image

- Each group now chooses to work with one of these episodes.
- Start with finding the most important moment in the story. Let those whose story it isn't offer their views first, and then hear the teller's view.

For health workers it is important to:

- really listen in this way, without too set an agenda of their own, balancing the specific things they may need to listen for with hearing what else is 'going on'

- recognise how revealing the patients' everyday stories are of who and how they are

- allow themselves to recognise their own versions of the basic dynamics contained in the stories they hear (*see also* Chapter 3 on narrative).

- The teller then acts as 'director' in setting up a still image of that moment, using the rest of the group as 'actors' in the roles involved, including that of the teller. It is a co-operative venture in which everyone may feel free to offer ideas, but the director has the final say. Directors stay out of the 'picture' but, if numbers dictate, may also be in it, preferably not as themselves.
- Set up the image in two different ways.

    1 **As if it were a photograph of the action** as it happened in reality. For this, pay attention to setting the scene. For example, if it is indoors, which room(s) are you in? Which bits of furniture are important enough to be in the scene? Where is the door, etc.? Set it clearly in space, using what is available, but only use what is really necessary to be clear.

    2 **As if it were a sculpt of the feelings and relationships** at that moment, picking up on the earlier sculpting idea. Show the relationship of 'characters' in 'space', using the space between them to express something about their relationship at that moment. Exaggerate body posture and facial expression appropriately.

- In both cases, animals and objects can be (and often are) 'characters'.
- Now, in either or both of them, what single word, or short phrase might each 'character' be saying in this moment? Actors offer ideas from within the roles, and the teller/director should adjust them if necessary. Then say the word or phrase.
- Perhaps show the rest of the group what each subgroup has done, without comment.
- Quick feedback, and then move on.

(ii) As three images

- Now choose someone else's scene. This time think of the event as having three key moments. As before, set up three still images as in 1 and/or 2 above, and give each character a phrase for each picture.
- Now find a way of moving from one picture to the next that preserves some theatrical formality and clarity and is not just a shuffle from one to the other.
- Show the images. In doing so, pay particular attention to starting and finishing. Wait at the beginning until everyone is still and silent, and then move into position. At the end, hold the picture still and silent for a moment, then make a formal break from it.

- *Note on timing:* Work quickly. This part of the session need take no longer that 20–30 minutes in total. Also, it is very important to think and discuss on your feet, working it out by trial and error rather than by protracted discussion. This also applies (especially) to the next part.

These pieces of work explore further what is going on, discovering how the episode unfolds, feeling the way physically into the dynamics of the relationships and what it is like to be the people in this story; and finding its shape, which then is given simple theatrical form.

Still images focus attention on the use of space – not only where people and things are in it at the chosen moment, but also how they relate to each other across it and what their bodies, caught in that moment, express. They sharpen our ability to notice the significant moment or gesture in whatever we experience – the moment and gesture that sum up the essence of it.

When the tellers speak in the first person as each of the 'characters' in their stories, except when they speak as themselves, even if they know the other characters well and heard what in reality they said, the words they choose will be more or less the fruit of intuition or intelligent guesses. All the more so for the other actors, whose only sense of the story is gained second-hand. Yet in a way the latter may be at an advantage. The story will almost certainly have a shape and pattern to it which they recognise from their own experience. They may well identify with the tellers. However, they may well also be able to identify with the other characters in the story, something the tellers may not be able to do as they are more likely bound up in their own point of view, needs and feelings. Their contributions may well therefore enable the tellers to see their stories in a different light, while nevertheless being true to the tellers' experience.

All of what has so far happened becomes much more active in the next stage of the work, namely the last act.

8 Mini productions

- Now either use the same story as in *6 Retelling the stories* above or choose another. This time the group will work towards a brief performance of the scene chosen (this is where break-out rooms are particularly useful).
- You can use any theatrical device you like within the limits of what is available. You have been working very physically up to now, but you can dialogue in either a 'realistic' convention or in a more stylised one, as you feel appropriate. The really

important thing is to be as true to the story and the teller's experience as possible, and to reveal the key elements of the story, the relationships and the feelings felt as clearly as possible. Use what we have been doing so far.

- Resist the temptation to invent things that didn't happen or to play it for laughs (or tears). If there is humour (or sadness) in it, of course you should reveal it, but let it speak for itself.
- On the other hand, in working on it, *do* risk intuiting what the 'characters' may be thinking and feeling, while checking these insights with the teller/director.
- Clearly, the dialogue and a good deal else, will be improvised and, apart from checking basic content and tone with the teller, will have to be left to the actors in performance.
- Allow no more than 40 minutes for creation and rehearsal, then bring everyone back together for each mini production to be performed. In the meantime, go from group to group now and then to check that they are not getting stuck and to help if they are. Or watch for a while and make suggestions if need be. Otherwise stay out of it and let them get on with it.
- Again, take care to set up each one properly and be clear about start and finish.
- See each in turn and then feed back what worked in each of them, and what was communicated.
- Then everyone can give feedback about the experience of doing it.
- This is where the 2- to 3-hour workshop ends.

EXAMPLES FROM WORKSHOPS

Some performances are sharper than others, and some subgroups struggle more than others, but their work has yielded a rich range of content and style and the process has been equally important to everybody.

Some of the scenes performed have been relatively lightweight, everyday episodes, such as getting stuck at the end of a queue in the post office. The teller was a little irritated at first, but soon just accepted his fate. He was able to observe what others were doing and what they seemed to feel. Not a big story you may think, in that he had little conflict to deal with and he coped very effectively with the event.

However, being at ease, he was able to observe how others were coping, and so the 'play' can reflect these others and offer actors the chance to inhabit those roles, which in turn will draw on their own experience of the feelings observed. Similarly, the play could celebrate the teller's own ease and what that means to him.

Yet the pattern of being stuck like this is very familiar. And it can produce a lot of emotional heat, although exactly how much will depend on the other pressures that are impinging on us. Given enough of them, the story of being stuck in the queue becomes as much the story of what is producing the pressures, our relationship with them and how we deal with them. We recognise it as a part of an archetypal story of our universal struggle with all the seemingly malevolent obstacles that block our progress through the day – life as an obstacle course! Most of the stories we have heard share something of this pattern, even if the emphasis turns out to be on something else.

That was what a working mother revealed in her episode, while juggling her children's needs with housekeeping and her husband, the car and getting to work. However, the key feeling to emerge was her sense of being a 'bad mother', which is in itself an obstacle, certainly, but is also more to do with the universal tension between caring for others and caring for ourselves.

Meanwhile, major life events happen with little respect for our daily routine. Another scene was 'set' in a possible new house, visited by the teller on the way to the workshop, and threw into relief the whole upheaval of thinking and feeling involved in her desire to move house. Another was a scene in the home of a patient who had died, and it involved giving support to the bereaved family.

Others reveal more cheerful moments – good news in the post, a tender moment between father and daughter, a grateful patient, and a hilarious meeting.

WORKING FROM PLAY TEXTS

So far we have started with personal experience and from it created 'plays', which could if we wished then be recorded and polished as texts. We shall now turn our attention to working from given texts.

Although it is an advantage to read a whole play before working on any part of it, for practical work it is easier and, for our purposes, more to the point to focus on short scenes of particular relevance. That way it doesn't take too much time to become familiar enough with the lines to get below the words to the experience of the characters involved. And that means being alive to the resonances it sets off in ourselves – what we share, even if only remotely, with them. For example, we may not have killed someone but we may well have felt like doing so and imagined doing it.

Thus exploring the given text by engaging physically and emotionally with the roles we are playing takes us into our own experience of the feelings and dilemmas felt by the characters, giving us a deeper sense both of ourselves and of what it might be like to 'be' them.

However, there is a big difference between just reading the words of a play text on the page and seeing it with a dramatic eye, finding the action in it, making visible and physical the feelings and relationships in three-dimensional space. Some playwrights help the actors with the action through stage directions. Others give no direction beyond the dialogue. This is why it is important to try acting them out. Before doing so, do some simple warm-up exercises described earlier in the chapter, or you can find others in a number of books available on the subject. Remember to pay attention to all the things suggested in the previous exercises. A few questions follow some extracts, of the kind that might help to reach through the text into the action.

Now try these scenes.

TWO SCENES FROM *SHADOWLANDS* BY WILLIAM NICHOLSON

In the 1950s, CS Lewis, the academic and author of the 'Narnia' books, is a confirmed bachelor, living a sheltered life in Oxford. Then, in his mid-fifties, he meets an admirer from America, a woman 20 years younger than him who is a prize-winning poet, highly intelligent and has a caustic wit. It is a meeting of like minds. They fall in love. Half of the play deals wittily with how he and his chauvinistic colleagues handle this disruption. But then the poet, Joy, develops bone cancer. In the second half the wit, and now the joy of love, is all the more poignant for the tragedy of illness, death and loss. Many of the scenes take place in the hospital. Joy has a remission and comes home with Lewis, and for a year they live happily together. Then the cancer takes hold again and she dies.

First scene

On one of his visits to the hospital Lewis talks with the doctor.

> **Doctor:** Well, Mr Lewis, I think I'm in no danger of overstating the case if I say, no news is good news. Given the seriousness of her condition, we have reason to be cautiously optimistic.

Lewis: I'm sorry, Doctor, but I don't understand a word you're saying. It would help me, if you would use words I'm familiar with, like 'getting better', 'getting worse'. 'Dying.'

Doctor: I'm afraid none of those words meet the case. What seems to be happening is that the rate of spread of the disease is slowing down.

Lewis: Is she better than she was?

Doctor: She's not worse.

Lewis: Is not-being-worse better than not-being-better.

Doctor: Put like that, yes.

Lewis: Thank you. Then she's better than she was.

Doctor: Mr Lewis. You're looking at a train, standing in a station. It may not be moving right now, but trains move. That's how trains are.

Lewis: What would be a good sign? People do recover from cancer. It has been known.

Doctor: Any sign of returning strength. Any sign that the body is rebuilding the diseased bone.

Lewis: Did you expect her to make it this far?

Doctor: What can I say? Remissions do happen.

(Lewis accepts this as the Doctor's attempt at encouragement)

Lewis: Thank you.

Both characters are struggling – the doctor with the reality of not knowing the answers, the difficulty of conveying this to Lewis, and dealing with Lewis's impatience and need for reassurance; Lewis with a desperate desire for Joy to be well, his need for simple yes/no answers, and his barely contained aggression.

The turning point in this brief encounter seems to be the doctor's graphic use of metaphor to convey the truth – or is it? And how will the doctor say those words? What is going on for him or her and how is it shown to the audience? How does the feeling reveal itself in action? How does Lewis's emotional state change in this scene?

Second scene

Lewis's wife has died. He is grief-stricken and has just attempted to re-enter his circle of friends for a drink, but was still too raw and angry. He has just left, having lost his temper with one of them. His brother, Warnie, follows him out.

Lewis: Sorry about that, Warnie. Not necessary.

Warnie: Everybody understands, Jack.

Lewis: I can't see her any more. I can't remember her face. What's happening to me?

Warnie: I expect it's shock.

Lewis: I'm so terribly afraid. Of never seeing her again. Of thinking that suffering is just suffering after all. No cause. No purpose. No pattern. No sense. Just pain, in a world of pain.

Warnie: I don't know what to say to you, Jack.

Lewis: Nothing. There's nothing to say.

They are silent for a few moments.

Douglas (Lewis's 8-year-old stepson) enters on the far side of the stage. He is profoundly hurt by his mother's death, but refusing to show it.

Warnie: Jack.

Lewis: Yes.

Warnie: About Douglas.

Lewis: Yes.

Warnie: Your grief is your business. Maybe you feel life is a mess. Maybe it is. But he's only a child.

Lewis: What am I supposed to do about it?

Warnie: Talk to him.

Lewis: I don't know what to say to him.

Warnie: Just talk to him.

You don't have to be a strong believer in an afterlife, as Lewis was, and to believe that suffering is God's way of sculpting us into more perfect human beings and so is part of His purpose and His gift to us, to feel the senselessness of it all, or the terror of not being able to 'see' her face any more (how does Lewis say, 'I can't remember her face'?); or the total self-absorption in grief and bewilderment that blinds him to the needs of others. Warnie has to shake him out of it, if only temporarily. How does Warnie say his final 'Talk to him'? Gently? Sharply?

Notice that the playwright gives Lewis the whole width of the stage to walk before he reaches Douglas. What for? And how might that be mirrored in your practice?

When he talks to Douglas it is, according to the stage directions, *'in a matter-of-fact way; as if they are equals'*, sharing the fact that his mother, too, died of cancer when he was eight and how that felt for him. Their brief conversation together and close contact unlock the tears that have so far refused to flow in either of them.

A SCENE FROM SHAKESPEARE'S MACBETH
(ACT 4, SCENE 3, LINE 159 ONWARDS)

Here we see in extraordinarily concentrated form the moment when Macduff hears of the murder of his wife and children at the hands of Macbeth. First, there is the poor messenger, Rosse, carrying the bad news. Like so many in his position, he really doesn't know how to handle it and desperately avoids the issue, even to the point when Macduff asks, 'How does my wife?' he answers cryptically, 'Why, well'.

Macduff: And all my children?

Rosse: Well too.

Macduff: The tyrant has not battr'd at their peace?

Rosse: No; they were well at peace, when I did leave 'em.

And when the news comes, it tumbles out in its starkest form. For a moment Macduff is shaken to the core, disorientated. The young Prince, Malcolm, leader of the armies resisting Macbeth, urges Macduff to convert his grief into action and revenge.

Malcom: Let's make us med'cines of our great revenge,

To cure this deadly grief.

Macduff: He has no children. – All my pretty ones?

Did you say all ? – O Hell-kite! –All?

What, all my pretty chickens, and their dam,

At one fell swoop?

Malcom: Dispute it like a man.

Macduff: I shall do so;

But I must also feel it as a man:

I cannot but remember such things were,

That were most precious to me. – Did Heaven look on,

And would not take their part? Sinful Macduff!

They were all struck for thee. Naught that I am,

Not for their own demerits, but for mine,

Fell slaughter on their souls: Heaven rest them now!

And so in a few lines he passes through disbelief, shock and grief, sweeps aside the younger man's urgings, and then goes on to railing against heaven and guilt at not being there to protect them and being the cause of their death. Then he puts off further mourning while he gets on with the war – and revenge. What are the key words in this and the other extracts that help bring out both sense and feeling – and, indeed, suggest action?

A SCENE FROM *SKIRMISHES* BY CATHERINE HAYES (PAGE 11)

Here is another death, but this time the focus is on the relationship between the two sisters meeting at their mother's bedside before she dies. Jean is the one who stayed with their mother and has looked after her all this time and Rita is the one who went away.

Jean: Did you bring me those cot sheets I asked for?

Rita: No, I didn't. I forgot.

Jean: I knew you would. You expect me to remember everything, though, don't you? If I forgot to send one of your brats a birthday card, I'd be the worst in the world. I buy the damn things in bulk now. Frankly, I've got them all written up for the next three years.

And, as so often happens, it is the absent daughter who is the mother's favourite:

Jean: She wants you, anyway. She's been waiting for you for weeks. Like before you were born. You were long overdue. She thought you'd never come. We were both waiting for you. And where were you? Nestled in the warm. Out of harm's way. Keeping us hanging on and hanging on. Knowing you'd arrive eventually, but not quite sure when …

And a bit later she says:

Jean: … Oh, God, I wish she'd hurry up and die. I want to do something else.

Even in such short extracts we encounter the bitterness of sibling rivalry and the usually silent wish for release through the parent's death. Most people would be able to access the feelings that go with the words to say them with vigour and conviction.

Similarly, the next extract deals with another mother/daughter relationship.

A SCENE FROM *MR WONDERFUL* BY JAMES ROBSON (ACT 1, SCENE 7)

This is a comedy with a sharply poignant edge. Norma's mother, Phoebe, has taken permanently to her bed, in the company of her teddy bear, Mr Wonderful, with whom she chats when otherwise alone. Norma is about 45 years old and unmarried. She has been dating men through an agency. The latest, Geoff, seemed different and the relationship was developing well, but her mother has intervened with a few well-placed lies about her daughter. The scene in which Norma confronts her mother ends like this:

Norma: This time, I thought it might different, this man, I thought – this man might love me as I need to be loved. He might really be tender and caring and bring me out of myself.

Phoebe: I'm sorry, Norma – really I am. *(She starts to snuffle, clutching Mr Wonderful to her bosom and dabbing her face with a tissue.)*

Norma: I was beginning to really like him. *(She turns to her mother.)* How could you hurt me like this?

(Phoebe wails and suddenly Norma is holding her.)

Phoebe: I could see that! I could see you'd clicked at last. I don't want to be left on my own!

(Shocked and staring, Norma moves on to the bed until she is sitting behind Phoebe and the old lady rests in her arms like a frail child. Phoebe snuffles and snuggles against her body.)

Phoebe: (Mumbling) Say you won't leave me, Norma, say you won't put me in a home. You're all I've got. I'm your mother.

(Norma looks down at her, still angry, but unable to speak)

Phoebe: Don't leave me, there's a good girl. What would I do? Norma …

(Norma stares down at Phoebe's face as her eyes close and the Light slowly closes in. Just before darkness gulps them down, Norma stares straight ahead as if numbed by the reality of her situation.)

Norma: (Murmuring) Mother.
(Blackout.)

Here we meet with betrayal, anger, disappointment, emotional blackmail, parent/child role reversal, love, the sense of duty and the terrible realisation of being trapped!

We have glimpsed here moments in just four very different texts whose action arises from illness and/or death, but which in their own different ways also throw into relief some common patterns in the way we relate to others. Not surprisingly, there are many plays that deal substantially with illness and death, all of which are of particular interest to the health professional. But the people you work with have plenty else to cope with in life – even happiness – and you can find plays that explore these things, too.

So, healthcare workers could usefully follow up the text work above by:

- identifying and playing scenes from their own experience
- practising ways of telling people bad news, or comforting people in distress, or whatever the play they are working with suggests, drawing from invented stories or directly from incidents in their own experience
- playing the recipient for others, so that they can experience what various approaches feel like and feeding that back
- imagining themselves into the scenes and helping the characters to resolve their differences or to handle their feelings
- making up scenes that explore such feelings and relationships
- playing as many of the different roles in such stories as possible to gain a better sense of how it feels to be in those shoes in those situations.

WHERE THE PLAYS MAY LEAD YOU

You may not yourself have experienced exactly what these characters have experienced, in the same circumstances or so extremely, although even Macduff's plight isn't all that unusual – but you will have experienced something with the same recognisable pattern, or hear in yourself an echo of it. There are many forms of loss, guilt, blackmail, inadequacy and joy. This is what you have to help your learners to access. No less important is what you have all already experienced in your imagination, through your hopes and fears, through your own 'as-if' explorations.

Many people find it easier to express their own emotions through the mouth of another. Playing the character may feel safer than playing ourselves and so may release the feelings in ourselves that resonate with those of the character. But now we can bring the feeling back into our own experience of it and explore it in the way described above.

CONCLUSION

Working through drama develops in us a sharper awareness of the following:

- the significance of apparently insignificant everyday events
- what it is like to 'be' other people
- the part that our physical self plays in that process
- the shape of events and their underlying patterns
- significant moments and gesture
- the importance of clarity and ways of achieving it through form and in space
- the potential of the dramatic process as an exploration of our experience
- how we communicate and negotiate in groups
- the usefulness of the activity for sharing experience and concerns with our peers and of being heard by them and supported – for what has been consistently demonstrated in this work is the care and respect with which participants treat each other and their stories
- the fun of group creativity.

It is with this last point this chapter ends – with the creative energy of laughter. Here is a task often used with groups of healthcare professionals that catches something of the playfully 'yah-boo' spirit of the game described earlier – 'There ain't no flies on us'. It also represents a whole area of work worth exploring further – creating your own fictions, thus bridging the gap between 'Working from personal experience' and 'Working from play texts'.

Being let loose

In groups of five take a half hour to create, for example, an advertising programme for recruiting staff and/or clients to the worst possible example of whatever organisation is appropriate to the group. It could be a clinic with a number of departments, thus giving a good spread of 'targets'. The idea is to sell all the worst examples of bad practice, real and imagined, as virtues, be they clinical, managerial, client care or type of client, thus sending up the system and saying the worst as exaggeratedly as possible. The structure could equally well be a mock documentary 'film' of, say, five scenes of everyday events there. While urging people to let their imaginations loose, it is useful to limit the number of 'scenes 'and to encourage shape and clarity in the presentation.

Group members will, of course, be drawing directly on their own experience, as all fiction does in one way or another, and the being let loose has, in my experience, been a release for worries and frustrations. But then the laughter usually clears a space for shared reflection. And there we are again – back to personal experience.

REFERENCES

Hayes C (1982) *Skirmishes*. Faber & Faber, London. pp. 11, 58–9.

Muir K (ed.) (1962) *'Macbeth' by William Shakespeare*. The Arden Edition, Methuen, London. pp 138–9.

Nicholson W (1992) *Shadowlands*. Samuel French, London. pp. 40 and 52–3.

Robson J (2000) *Mr Wonderful*. Samuel French, London. pp. 39–40.

PART II

INTRODUCTION

Part II is about 'what happened next', as what we shall describe in this part is some of the teaching work we have undertaken since writing the first edition of this book. Much of this teaching was in response to the curriculum for specialty training for general practice training introduced by the Royal College of General Practitioners in the UK in 2006, which attempts to prepare doctors not just with good scientific knowledge and communication skills but also with a global understanding of the patient within the family and society, and how this relates to good medical practice.

We have continued to learn about and to observe the contribution the arts can make in teaching, and to discover wonderful new resources. This is about developing and expanding the resources we use.

In Part I we invited you to come on a journey. We now want to give you the confidence to visit and explore new territories, and while there to have the courage to see what might be beyond the horizon.

Part II

10 THINKING IT THROUGH

1 THE HOLISTIC APPROACH

How do you teach holistic care?

This is a question that we have been asked – with the implied query 'might using the arts be a good way?'.

Understanding a patient's life, ideas and mythologies is an essential start to a holistic approach. An important part of healthcare is interpreting illness in the context of the individual, and their family, community and culture. Appropriate therapies and interventions are often an agreed management plan that takes into account adopting patients' perspectives, knowing something about their environment and expectations. The ability to listen and respond to a patient's narrative, to tolerate ambiguity, and to recognise the meanings of events will help communication. Relevant scientific knowledge is vital in treating patients. Comprehending their experience of illness is just as necessary.

How do you gain skills to work in this way?

The arts are a good way of learning about people. The skill of the artists is in transporting us to places and allowing us to experience events possibly outside our own world – to understand, gain empathy and realise our own limitations.

A teaching session needs to use resources which will engage learners in this process, followed by facilitation of their responses and a discussion of the practical application in medical work.

Here is an example of a work plan.

Work plan

Start with art.

Aim

The aim is to gain understanding of how we explain and give meaning to things and events.

Resource

The resource is a collection of reproductions (e.g. postcards) spread out on a table, showing a variety of subjects – landscape, portraits, events and abstract images.

> Ask your group to look at the images. Then ask each learner to choose one to take from the table and to sit down with a neighbour and tell each other about the card they have chosen. (If two people want the same card, they can discuss it or one give way and choose another card.) Then display the selected cards all together and discuss them as a group.

What happens

Group members will have noticed and given priority to or rejected different things in the images, despite them all looking at the same material. They will have expressed quite definite feelings and ideas when informing their neighbour about their choice. The collection of selected images will be an interesting reflection of the group's preferences.

Facilitation

The group will be able to see that they have selected differently, but they will have shared their observations, ideas and intuitions and may have gained extra knowledge and experience. Ask them to consider the language – finding the right words – they used to explain their choice of image. For example, did they use metaphor, or 'it reminded me of'? What were the connections between the image and their previous experience and feelings and what they really wanted to communicate to each other?

Next relate this to the consultation and discuss how a patient may try to describe/explain from their own memory images and feelings – what has happened to them – hoping that you will listen and understand.

Follow this with some work aimed at understanding the experience of illness and how it affects people's lives, and the related dilemmas and problems of medical staff.

Suggested resources

Literature which has a medical theme, such as the following.

• *Regeneration* by Pat Barker (*see* page 34).

- *Saturday* by Ian McEwan. A neurosurgeon's conflict with a patient who has Huntington's Chorea – the effects on the surgeon's family.
- *The Secret Scripture* by Sebastian Barry. Set in Ireland, this is the narrative of a patient and the doctor who treats her.
- *The Last Town on Earth* by Thomas Mullen. A town that tries to isolate itself from an epidemic with resulting tragedies, and dilemmas and problems for medical staff.
- *Face*, a short story by Alice Munro about a child born with a birthmark.
- *Outpatients*, a poem by Carole Satyamurti (*see* page 48).

> Get the group members to read the text you have chosen as homework.
>
> Ask them to document what they think the story is about, what it made them feel, what they were reminded of, and how it connected to their medical work.

Facilitation

Discuss the group's responses, aiming to validate any intuitions and observations about illness in communities, the effect of environment, the patient's experience as narrated, and the way a doctor may learn from what happens, to change behaviour.

Other resources

Use a film clip as well (*see* Chapter 8, 'Take one: teaching with film'), perhaps from *The Death of Mr Lasarescu*, a Czech film about a patient who is shunted from hospital to hospital, and has great difficulty in having his condition appreciated and treated, with some good and bad communication and care. Facilitate responses as above.

End the session with an open discussion. Get group members to reflect on the following.
- What did I learn?
- What will I do differently in future?
- Have I identified any further learning needs?

2 How do I look?
Face to face with self-portraits

'Every painter paints himself.'

Michelangelo

An essential part of the diagnosis and treatment of disease is the medical image – X-ray pictures, CT and MRI scans – which show the inside of the body in order to confirm normality or identify abnormality.

It is easy for these images to be regarded as 'the patient' without valuing how we actually see the whole patient and relate to and understand that person in their human context.

The consultation is a two-way process – the doctor or nurse sees the patient, but the patient also sees the doctor or nurse. What visual information does each gather?

Patients express a strong desire to communicate, to convey their personal circumstances, to establish their identity. The doctor or nurse also wants to establish an identity.

We suggest that using self-portraits can be a good tool to use in work aiming to give insight into how people choose to represent themselves and how they are seen – on both sides of the consultation desk.

What are the features of self-portraits? *(Several examples were given in Part I – Jenny Saville and Munch – but Goya's self-portrait with Dr Arrieta might be good to show.)*

A self-portrait is rarely a straight mirror image. Artists paint themselves with friends and family, in a particular environment, sometimes in a different role or in the presence of those they admire or aspire to. They paint themselves at different times in their lives – youthful or ageing. They try to capture how they are when ill, from both physical and psychological causes. It is a question of identity – 'This is who I am, this is how I feel'.

Resource
Paintings in *500 Self Portraits* Phaidon Press.

Ask each learner to select a painting and talk about it.

- How is the artist wanting to be seen?
- How do I see it?
- How does this affect me?
- What have I learnt about the person in the painting?

Facilitation
Facilitate responses with group discussion. When everyone in the group has had a turn, look at the selection of paintings chosen,

and establish what the differences are and how much information has been gathered.

Or, as an alternative, show the same painting(s) to everyone and invite their responses as above.

You will find that everyone will have different responses to looking at the same painting. Discuss the relevance of this.

CREATE YOU OWN SELF-PORTRAIT

If you have a group with whom you are working over a period of time, and have the opportunity to give them homework between sessions, ask the learners to produce their own self-portraits. This can be done in any medium (including photography) of their choice.

Precede this exercise with work about image, as described above and in Chapter 6.

What does this exercise achieve?

Group members will produce portraits which attempt to present something about themselves that they are prepared to share, and to explain their representation of self in everyday working life. Here are some examples.

- A collage of the doctor's face, to convey the 'mask' we put on as doctors. The collage was made from torn-up pieces of medical publications and the colours were very important in emphasising different parts of the face (eyes, ears, mouth) used in the consultation. The student had enjoyed the process of creating this picture, first by fragmentation and then by reconstitution.
- A photo of the doctor's head in the middle of the page, surrounded by eight photographed hands, juggling different jobs – shown as symbolic words – empowering patients, money, rationing, targets, etc. Some of the letters were falling off the edge of the picture, and in the background was a huge prescription pad.
- A drawing of the student (a medical educator) transposed as a sheet of lightning hitting the ground – an image rich in metaphor for:
  - work – lightning only strikes where something comes up from the earth
  - education – is not just about giving information, but receptors must also be put out, and then ideas can be sparked.

3 DIVERSITY AND EQUALITY

A holistic approach also values diversity and equality by recognising and valuing difference, by attempting to be part of a fair society, and by using opportunities to fulfil patients' needs in a non-judgmental and open way – with good communication skills.

We suggest that the use of arts resources in teaching can be appropriate and helpful in achieving understanding in this area.

Artists and photographers have observed, captured and recorded humanity in all its aspects. In literature, writers have told stories about events and the relationships of people, based in many different cultures and environments, which can invoke our emotions and feelings. These can all help to clarify our understanding of the concept of diversity and equality.

EXERCISES
Try using texts

Use texts that have doctors as the main characters, and set in different cultures. For example, *The Good Doctor* by Damon Galgut concerns South Africa. The first chapter alone is a good basis for discussion as it describes a young doctor who starts work in an unfamiliar environment and feels overwhelmed by all the issues he will have to understand.

Create a presentation

Prepare a presentation showing a series of paintings and photographs which illustrate humanity in all its guises. Look for images which show traditional representations of family and relationships and contrast these with those that are different and show other aspects of life. Find portraits from:

- other cultures
- from history (e.g. events where human beings have undergone deprivation, loss and misunderstanding contrasted with images of privilege)
- scenes which highlight differences between rural and urban life.

Show your presentation

Show your presentation to the group as a slide show, without any commentary, asking learners to note any image that has some significance for them.

Facilitate a discussion where group members talk about these images, bringing them back up on the screen as appropriate. Note any issues that might need further clarification and those where there may have been disagreement – an alternative view.

An alternative in this exercise of creating your own programme is to ask your group members in advance to find and bring their own images – ones that for them say something about diversity. Be sure to have a well thought out strategy for how you will combine and show everyone's contributions. Advise the learners to spend some time finding their images, not just to look the night before the session! You may find that some group members are unsure about what they need to do and may not contribute. This in itself may say something about their difficulties in coping with diversity in their professional lives.

Show a film clip

Have a clear aim about what you want to achieve in choosing your film.

See 'The Diving Bell and the Butterfly' in Chapter 11 for a detailed discussion about using clips from this film to teach about diversity and equality.

Any facilitation of discussion should aim to help learners to increase their awareness of preconceptions.

To avoid stereotyping, it is important to understand the differences between people, to have good communication skills and always to be prepared to learn and reflect on new knowledge about patients' experiences and lives. Empathy means being able to put yourself in the same place as the other person – it means that you know what it feels like.

4 FINDING THE RIGHT WORDS

Many doctors and nurses choose to work away from their country of origin, and need to consult in a language other than their own first language. Medical educators may find themselves teaching English language to international medical graduates and medical students from other countries. This teaching is not just about demonstrating the use of vocabulary, but should also help students to comprehend nuance, hidden agendas, the use of metaphor and phrases used in negotiation strategies, and to respond appropriately.

How can educators acquire the skills for this?

Here is an exercise whose aim is to enable educators to practise finding the right words and understanding the words of others in a situation which is new to them.

Resource

Laminates, A6-size of paintings of your choice (e.g. showing medical scenes or self-portraits).

> Divide the learners into groups of three and give a painting at random to each group.
>
> Ask each group to discuss their painting among themselves. What do they see? What do they feel? What does it connect with in their experience?
>
> Each group should then present their painting to the rest of the learners – succinctly and capturing the essence of it.
>
> The facilitator will take note of phrases and vocabulary used, and be prepared to ask why they are being used, whether there are alternatives, what words would other learners have used, and what is their understanding?

How does it work?

In this exercise, the situation is outside everybody's normal work. Everyone can feel equal and not constrained – there is no hierarchy of knowledge. The paintings and their narratives are the common point. The mechanisms involved in self-expression – in particular the words and phrases used to describe, to relay emotion, to talk about past events, and convey this to others in a manner that is understood and invites reciprocal communication – will be demonstrated.

Suggest to the educators that they then repeat this exercise with their foreign students. Include a full discussion at the end, in which the students address the following.

• What did I learn?
• How can I apply this?
• What more do I need to do to reinforce this learning?

5 SIGNIFICANT EVENTS – EVERYDAY DRAMAS?

Reflecting on and writing up significant events which occur in the daily working life is an essential requirement in a trainee's educational portfolio, and later for professional appraisal and revalidation.

What are the characteristics of such events? What is their effect? Consider the following.

- Significant events have many players – those featuring in the action, those who are coincidental observers, and those who have to resolve or find solutions to the event.
- Patient narratives are a collection of significant events which they want to talk about –what do they choose to tell and how (often with imagery and metaphor).
- Significant events can cause/induce change. How is this coped with? What influences the process? What is learnt?

Art, literature and film are resources for looking at representation, description and enactment of significant events. Using such resources can be a way in which to help people understand their own observations and feelings – what they identify with and how they make decisions when dealing with significant events.

TEACHING SESSION
Aim
- To examine the experience of being part of a significant event.
- To discuss the structure of significant event analysis and how to record events.

Resource
A Small Good Thing, a short story by Raymond Carver.

Ask your group to read the story in advance.

The story recounts a hit and run accident involving a child on his birthday – how his parents cope, the child's medical care, and what happens to a baker, commissioned to make a birthday cake for the child.

Divide your group into pairs. Ask them to identify the main players in the story and those characters who are incidental to the main action, and which ones have to resolve or find a solution to the event.

Allocate a main player (character) to each pair. They are coming to see their GP. Ask each pair to consider the issues their character will have, and how the GP will manage them.

Ask each pair in turn to present their work, either as role play or as a simple account of their ideas, to the rest of the group.

Facilitation

Document the issues that the pairs identify, also asking for additional insights which occur to other members of the group as the exercise progresses.

Discuss how the group members arrived at their thoughts through having used the material given to them by the author in the story. What intuitions, and in particular what feelings, were engendered by the writer's ability to make the events cohesive, understandable, informative and humane? The discussion might also include ideas on how the author has chosen to construct the narrative. What changes happened to characters because of the events?

> Ask the group members to document the significant event as if they were the doctor in the story and then to share their writing with the rest of the group.

Facilitation

Discussion about the ways of writing up significant events may be necessary at this point. The Gibbs reflective cycle is a useful model to use – this is involves six stages.

1 What happened?
2 What were you thinking or feeling?
3 What was good or bad about the experience?
4 What sense could you make of the situation?
5 What else could you have done?
6 If the situation arose again, what would you do?

GP trainees in the UK may prefer to follow headings in their eportfolio template.

* What happened?
* What issues were raised?
* What was done well?
* What was not done well?
* What could be done differently in the future?
* What (personal) learning needs did you identify?
* How and when will you address these?

Discuss what has been learnt. Flag up areas of further learning needs.

Allow time at the end of your session for anyone to discuss a significant event from their own life that is on their mind and, as a result of what has been discussed, has acquired some insight or anxiety about it.

6 UNDERSTANDING OLD AGE

As the proportion of older people in society increases, the importance of understanding old age and the process of ageing is becoming more important. It is one of the curriculum topics which UK trainee GPs have to study. For many young medical professionals old age is something to be endured in the dim and distant future – few consider what it is like to be old, but for some there may be painful experiences around health problems in an old relative.

Arts resources are a powerful tool to help trainees engage with questions such as the following.

- What does it really feel like to be old?
- What do older people think about?
- What is their perception about what is happening to them?

Medical texts can help with understanding the pathophysiology of the ageing process which occurs in various parts of the body (e.g. the brain in dementia). There are clear descriptions of how the condition is manifest and what changes in behaviour and other brain functions lead to the diagnosis.

But this is not the whole story for the person who is growing old. There is something beyond the medical textbooks which is to do with the person. Here is the outline of a teaching session with a group of GP trainees, which we believe gives them a more holistic approach to the understanding of old age. It acknowledges objective scientific explanations of the process of ageing, but also explores the idea that people have inner experiences which are subjective and which affect their health and health beliefs.

Aim
- To see old age from the patient's point of view (empathy).
- To encourage a holistic approach to the problems presented by ageing.

Start by asking the learners to define old age (the answer apparently lies anywhere between 60 and 80!).

Facilitation

Quiz each learner and ask for the rationale behind their answer. Use a flip chart to make a bar chart of the frequency of chosen age. This is a non-threatening way to begin to explore the learners' preconceptions.

> Continue within the learners' medical comfort zone and ask them to discuss in small groups what exactly ageing is and why it occurs.

Facilitation

This provides an opportunity to explore the limitations and relevance of scientific knowledge.

> Next, ask the learners to describe an old person in their lives – this might be a relative, a family friend, a patient or a character from the media or literature. Initially, the learners should work in pairs, and then the whole group can share the results.

Facilitation

Explore what this person has meant to them and why. Encourage the learners to start discussing their feelings.

> The next challenge for the learners is to disclose the words or phrases that first came to mind when they heard the phrase 'old person', and why. Put these onto the flip chart.

Facilitation

Use the words to start the group thinking widely around the concepts and stereotypes of old age. Encourage the learners to consider positive images and concepts (e.g. wisdom, kindness, experience and interesting stories) as well as negative ones (e.g. loneliness, incontinence, deafness, cognitive impairment and depression).

As discussed in the Chapter 6, 'A way of seeing', we all have different abilities in conjuring up a visual image. However, artists are experts at observing, capturing and recording the essence of what they see.

So to help those learners who have difficulty in conjuring up an image of an old person in Exercises 3 and 4, the exercise can be enhanced by showing the picture *Last Sickness* by Alice Neel (*see* page 82), and asking the following fundamental questions.

- What do you see? (By this we mean everything about the picture – her facial expression, surroundings, hands, hair, dressing gown. etc.)
- What does it make you feel? (Broaden that out into feelings about being asked to visit residential and nursing homes.)
- How do you respond? (Considering yourself as both self and a doctor.)

> Watch a recording of Alan Bennett's monologue *A Cream Cracker under the Settee*, in which an old lady, Doris, falls in her flat and almost certainly sustains a hip fracture. The monologue is a moving narrative of her immediate circumstances and her likely future (fear of going to hospital and then into care), together with her reflections about the challenges she has encountered in her life.

Facilitation

Follow the 'rules' for showing films:

- watch
- allow time for reflection and re-integration into present reality
- start a discussion.

Divide the learners into three groups to discuss what they have just seen, and what their feelings and responses were. Try to get them to imagine themselves in Doris's predicament and to think about her emotions – in pain, only able to move with difficulty, and fearful about an uncertain future. Try to get them to understand that she is constructing a new narrative which is interwoven with events from her life (the importance of what is remembered) and her reaction to them, which, one comes to realise, inform how she is coping with her sudden new predicament. This will involve the learners in thinking about empathy and the nature of the patient narrative.

This piece of learning can be reinforced by constructing three scenarios for them to role play:

- the confrontation between Doris and a social worker trying to persuade her to go into residential care
- the likely consultation between Doris and her GP, who had been called to see her following her fall

- a conversation between Doris and her orthopaedic consultant following hip surgery.

Encourage the group to use all their imaginative and creative skills and enable them to see how the insights they have gain from their work in Exercises 1–4 on constructing the patient's point of view have informed the vignettes they have constructed, and how these may be ignored by the health professionals involved in Doris's care. This final exercise should emphasise the importance of empathy in effective communication.

11 DESTINATIONS

1 THE DIVING BELL AND THE BUTTERFLY

The Diving Bell and the Butterfly is a book by Jean-Dominique Bauby, which has been made into a film directed by Julian Schnabel, the winner of a Cannes Festival Golden Globe.

We shall illustrate how a resource can be used as a tool in teaching many parts of the curriculum, including those described in earlier chapters.

This book, and the film of the book, is a true story – an account by a patient, once a celebrity editor of *Elle* magazine, of his experience after a stroke. The stroke caused locked-in syndrome, and left him able to see and hear normally, but physically paralysed – not able to talk, only able to blink an eyelid. Throughout the film, it is his thoughts that we hear, superimposed on scenes in the hospital, and re-enacted flashbacks of his life before the stroke. The original book was dictated by him to a speech therapist, who had devised a method of interpreting his eye blink sequence in relation to the alphabet to create words.

Here are some of the topics where you could use this resource in teaching.

DISABILITY

Although physically disabled, the patient is able to think, see, hear, use his imagination and draw upon his memory. However, the film illustrates the frustration of not being able to communicate in the usual way. We see through his eyes how people react to him – for example, the telephone engineers who come into his hospital room, and their inability to know what to say, resorting to misplaced humour to cover their embarrassment.

We understand through the patient's commentary what it feels like suddenly to be unable to do normal things and to have to find a way of adapting to this state in order to cope with life as it now is, and to battle with depression, hopelessness and fear.

Give your learners the following exercise to do, which mimics the method Jean-Dominique used to communicate.

> In this exercise the learners should communicate without speaking or using any facial expression – only using blinking an eyelid.
>
> Divide the group into pairs, with one of the pair as the doctor, the other as the patient. Give each *patient* a slip of paper with the message '*I think I am getting side-effects from the medication*' written on it. Tell them that this thought has to be communicated to their doctor (who must not see it in writing).
>
> The *doctor* must tell their patient that in order to get the message they will speak the alphabet (a, b, c, d …) and ask their patient to blink when they get to the letter that is needed to make the words of the message. The doctor should write down each letter, and read out the message when it has been understood.

Facilitation

Get everyone to talk about what it felt like to do this task – for both the *patient* and the *doctor*. They will talk about frustration, impatience, irritation, feeling helpless, stupid and incompetent, wanting to improvise and invent, the realisation of how much we take for granted until suddenly it isn't there, and the need for empathy and tolerance. Discuss in this teaching about disability– the importance of understanding the experience of illness as a patient, and not as the doctor concentrating on causation and treatment alone.

COMMUNICATION SKILLS

At the beginning of the film, the patient is seen coming out of the fog of unconsciousness, and we hear his thoughts as he attempts to comprehend where he is and what is happening. We understand his frustration at not being able to communicate and having to rely on everything being said to him for information, but not able to ask questions or to show any positive or negative response, or to tell anyone of his fear.

We see the medical staff at his bedside and hear the consultant talking to him. Later, we see the insensitive approach by an ophthalmologist attempting to work on his eyelid.

Exercise to look at communication skills involved in a one-way situation

Get the group to comment on how the doctors communicate in the film as above, with reference to the information and the way it is delivered – in particular to the statement by the doctor to the patient that 'Your condition is very rare'. Ask how much of what is said is the doctor's agenda and how much is the patient's.

Next, divide the group into pairs, with a doctor and a patient (who is unable to respond) in each pair. Decide on a medical condition for the patient, and ask the doctor to talk to the patient about it.

Facilitation

Discuss how the doctor decided what he would say, and then ask if the patient thought that what was said was acceptable. Talk about alternative ways of giving information effectively. What criteria are involved? Ask the patients what they would have said if they had been able to respond. From this discussion formulate some guidelines which as teachers you could give to students to use when talking to an apparently unresponsive patient.

Uses of imagery

The two things Jean-Dominique Bauby says he can still use are his imagination and his memory. In the film, there are specific images to show us this in practice. In reading the book we would form our own images from his written thoughts. It is worth discussing with the group how awareness of our own imagination – how we activate it and harness the results in communication – could help to get into the world of a sick patient whose needs we are attempting to understand.

Cinematic imagery is used at the beginning of the film to try to convey what the *patient* is experiencing, with deliberate fuzziness and incomplete frames. We also see flashing X-ray images and a kaleidoscope of medical pictures of what is happening to the patient – what *doctors* will need to know to diagnose, treat and manage him effectively. It is important to acknowledge *both* these sets of images.

NARRATIVE MEDICINE

The action in the film goes back and forth from present, as in the consultation. Events being drawn from the patient's memory are interspersed with the live happenings. It is necessary for the observer or reader to make sense of all of this and understand the whole, seeing where each bit fits in and has influence on the present.

Get your learners to comment on this and draw parallels with their own experience in hearing and telling stories.

UNDERSTANDING RELATIONSHIPS – HOLISTIC CARE

A patient's illness and dilemma affects their relationships with their family and friends, and this often involves medical staff who may have to help and advise.

Staff in a medical unit often have no prior knowledge of a patient's pre-morbid personality or traits, and just see and relate to the patient as he or she is in his or her illness state. In the film, we see how, when communication is limited, the dominance is with the able-bodied, and does not take into account the other side of the patient's personality – now hidden, but shown in cinematic flashbacks from his memory.

This illustrates the importance in holistic care of getting as wide an understanding of all aspects of a patient as possible, rather than basing care only on a superficial inventory of symptoms and test results.

In the film, the speech therapist is a real star. She does not give up when confronted with non-engagement from her patient and challenges and examines both her professional role and the patient's negativity. She thinks through both her own agenda and the patient's responses, and with courage finds a solution to communication which revolutionises the patient's psychological recovery and enables him to start being able to record and express his story.

We see poignancy and distress in the relationship between the patient and his elderly father, now having to cope with a new way of relating to each other as their roles are in some way reversed. A flashback shows Jean-Dominique treating his father as a helpless, childlike figure when he is having to shave him. Then a photograph is shown of Jean-Dominique as a child with his strong father – the patient now feels back in that dependent state.

Those who knew Jean-Dominique well now see him in a changed physical state and have to manage their reactions and feelings. We are conscious of how the patient perceives this and has to find an inner way of coping with this changed response from them.

2 KING LEAR

In Chapter 9, 'The drama of everyday life', David Powley discussed how drama can heighten our awareness of:

- the significance of apparently insignificant everyday events (*narrative*)
- what it is like to 'be' other people (*empathy*)
- the shape of events and their underlying patterns (*narrative*)
- significant moments and gestures (*cues*)
- the importance of clarity and ways of achieving it through form and in space (*communication skills*)
- the potential of the drama process as an exploration of our experience (*holism*)
- how we communicate and negotiate in groups (*communication skills*).

You will see that many of these subheadings form an important part of any medical curriculum.

We next describe a theatre visit with GP trainees to see *King Lear* by Shakespeare, which again demonstrates the relevance of drama in medical education.

The *aims* for the exercise were laid out in the following briefing given to students before the trip:

> I expect you will be asking: what on earth has a Shakespeare play to do with GP training? Well, apart from a theatre visit being enjoyable in its own right, consider how you yourselves and your patients are actors, reacting in very different ways in different circumstances. Reflect on Shakespeare's amazing insights into human behaviour, how he analyses and portrays all the great themes of life (and death). Ponder on the language used in the play and how difficult it is sometimes to follow the logical thread in an argument on stage and how this can happen when you are consulting, especially if the patient uses words you don't understand and metaphors you haven't come across before.
>
> I would like you to reflect on the themes, motives and symbols in this brutal play. Here are a few clues to get you thinking.
>
> - How does Shakespeare portray the problems of old age? How does this relate to the reality you see?
> - How are trust and betrayal explored? Have you seen parallels in your personal and professional life?
> - What was difficult about the language used in the play? Are there similarities with the consultation?

The following week we looked at what we had learnt from the play.

> Introduce a general discussion between groups of two or three
> trainees about the play, in terms of:
>
> • language and communication
> • old age
> • mental health and in particular dementia
> • human relationships, emotions and behaviour, and death
>   and dying
> • the drama of life and the part we play as actors.

Facilitation

Each pair or trio then bring their thoughts to the whole group for discussion. It is a good idea to have prepared your own thoughts in advance about each example heading for dementia:

• the early inability of Lear accurately to sum up what was happening and his misuse of power
• his difficulty in comprehension and confabulation to explain things
• his disinhibition
• his loss of contact with reality
• his regression to infantile behaviour.

> The trainees were then asked to think how the description
> of dementia in a standard psychiatry textbook (ask them to
> look at this as pre-course work) might compare with the way
> Shakespeare depicts it in the play – has Shakespeare helped
> them to understand what really happens when a family
> member becomes demented, and if so what is that reality?

> The GP's role is often to mediate. The GP may be the only
> person who is common to all sides and can give help without
> emotional involvement. The play shows how old people can be
> taken advantage of, despatched to care homes and stripped
> of their possessions and dignity without consultation. GPs are
> often involved in consultations when the question of power
> of attorney is under discussion. Distress and dissent within
> the involved families can sometimes result in psychosomatic
> illness, which presents to the GP.

> Devise a consultation where Cordelia, Goneril, Reagan and
> her husband have gone to their GP to discuss Lear's changing
> mood and mental state and want power of attorney. Ask
> trainees to role play the consultation.

Facilitation

Bring into the discussion the issues for the family and the GP. What
are the family relationships portrayed in the play and how might
different family members react?

WHAT HAPPENED

The reaction of the trainees to this experience was generally very
positive. One wrote 'it was a fun way of exploring and reflecting
on instances we have had in consultations with patients and their
families along with the emotions they evoke'.

3 SCULPTURE REVISITED

In Chapter 7 we introduced you to the Yorkshire Sculpture Park
(YSP) as an example of a location which had the power to inspire,
to take us out of ourselves and encourage us to view the world
from a different perspective. We briefly described a simple task for
trainees to try and their responses to the experience.

We would now like to take you back there to explore the
diversity of themes which might inspire creative medical teaching.
(The experience is not unique to the YSP and could be achieved
at any major art installation.) Some of these themes are generic
and may not seem immediately to relate to any specific medical
(curriculum) topic.

The following are possible learning outcomes.

- Experiencing group learning in a different environment – many
  people have no experience of sculpture and find it a challenging
  art form which may be way beyond their comfort zone. If you
  are having difficulty and wondering how this relates to medical
  practice, consider that many patient encounters may take place
  outside the comfort and familiarity of the GP's consulting room
  or the hospital ward.
- Exploring the educational and professional challenges of ambiguity and hidden meanings. In many aspects of medical practice
  all may not be what it seems. One of the skills of the healthcare
  professional is to interpret the often strange and non-linear

narratives which patients construct, the examination findings which do not fit with the diagnosis, and the investigation and imaging results which appear to be at odds with the diagnosis. All of these relate to ambiguity, which must be learnt about. There are many parallels here with sculptures – their complex and often abstract forms making an ideal substrate for conversation and discussion.

- An opportunity to think in terms of metaphors (we have already considered this through poetry in Chapter 4, 'The language of feelings') for everyday practice, especially in the interpretation of visual images.
  - What is the sculptor (patient) trying to tell you?
  - What do the sculptures (patients) make you feel?
  - How do you respond and why?
- Think how tactile information has been relegated within the practice of medicine. Much less emphasis is now placed on the physical examination of the patient – much of the information previously gained through the hands of the physician is now obtained using technology. Many different materials are used for sculpture and this produces different surfaces and textures to be experienced. This is a good opportunity to start discussions about the role of hands in our interactions with patients.
- Unlocking creativity. How can this be achieved?
  - By giving groups digital cameras to record a narrative of their experience and their learning. The images may be of the sculptures themselves or of their interaction with them. Free licence and encouragement is given to be creative in this task. The sculptures are just a starting point for this creative task. The digital narrative is presented when the groups meet to discuss their experiences.
  - One of the exhibits at the YSP is a collection of mesostic poems by Alec Finlay. These poems are in the form of labels naming plants and have a name-stem and word-branches:

NAMES
MAKE
STEMS
CHOSEN
WORDS
THEIR
GROWING
BRANCHES

The challenge for learners was to create their own mesostic poems around words connected with education and training. The exercise inspired the following poem.

C**R**EATIVITY
A**DD**RESSES
S**U**BTLE
DEFI**C**IENCIES
ENCOU**RA**GING
UNDERS**T**ANDING
INSP**I**RING
J**O**Y
K**N**OWLEDGE

ACKNOWLEDGEMENTS

The authors and publishers gratefully acknowledge the following individuals and organisations for their permission to reproduce the images and extracts used in this book.

CHAPTER 1

- Jonathan Wyatt (ed.) (1999) The Oxford Handbook of Accident and Emergency Medicine. OUP. By permission of Oxford University Press.
- Sebastian Junger (1997) The Perfect Storm. Reprinted by permission of HarperCollins Publishers Ltd. © 1997 Sebastian Junger.
- The Lady In the Van by Alan Bennet (© 1989 Forelake Ltd) is used by permission of United Agents (www.unitedagents.co.uk) on behalf of Forelake Ltd.
- Schumann Piano Works CD cover. Courtesy of Naxos.
- Steep Lane Baptist Church, Yorkshire (1976) © Martin Parr/Magnum Photos. By permission of Magnum Photos.

CHAPTER 3

- Véronique Mistiaen's Life after a Mastectomy, published in The Times Magazine.
- Roddy Doyle (1996) The Woman Who Walked into Doors. Jonathan Cape. Reprinted by permission of The Random House Group.
- From REGENERATION by Pat barker, © 1991 by Pat Barker. Used by permission of Dutton Signet, a division of Penguin Group (USA) Inc.
- Spending Time (1986) © Martin Parr/Magnum Photos. By permission of Magnum Photos.

Chapter 4

- Virginia Woolf's On Being Ill. The Society of Authors as the Literary Representative of the Estate of Virginia Woolf.
- RS Thomas (2004) Collected Later Poems, 1998–2000. Bloodaxe Books.
- 'Musée des Beaux Arts' Copyright © 1940 by WH Auden and renewed. Reprinted by permission of Curtis Brown, Ltd.
- 'Changing the subject'. From Selected Poems (2000) by Carole Satyamurti, published by Bloodaxe Books.
- 'Across the border' © Karen Fiser. From Words Like Fate and Pain (1992) by Karen Fiser, published by Zoland Press. Reproduced with permission of the copyright holder.
- Reprinted by permission of the publishers and the Trustees of Amherst College from THE POEMS OF EMILY DICKINSON, Thomas H Johnson ed., Cambridge, Mass.: The Belknap Press of Harvard University Press, Copyright © 1951, 1955, 1979, 1983 by the President and Fellows of Harvard College.
- 'The Old Fools' from COLLECTED POEMS by Philip Larkin. Copyright © 1988, 2003 by the Estate of Philip Larkin. Reprinted by permission of Farrar, Straus and Giroux, LLC.
- Susan Spady's 'Flower leaning from a vase', published by Blue Heron Press.
- 'The handicapped'. From Night Shift at the Crucifix Factory (1991) by Philip Dacey, published by the University of Iowa Press. Reproduced with permission of the copyright holder.
- Sophie Large's 'Sunglasses', published by the Trustees of Sophie's Silver Lining Fund, www.sslf.org.uk
- THE QUARREL by Conrad Aiken. Copyright © 1929, 1956 by Conrad Aiken. Used by permission of Brandt and Hockman Literary Agents, Inc. Any copying or distribution of this text is expressly forbidden. All rights reserved.
- TS Eliot's 'Burnt Norton'. From the 'Four Quartets', in Collected Poems 1909–1962 by TS Eliot. Used by permission of Faber & Faber Ltd. © 1936 Harcourt Inc., renewed 1964 by TS Eliot.

Chapter 6

- Rooms by the Sea (1951), by Edward Hopper. © Yale University Art Gallery, Bequest of Stephen Carlton Clark BA, 1903.
- The Subway (1950), by George Tooker. © Reproduction rights granted by DC Moore Gallery, New York, on behalf of the artist.

- Mr and Mrs Clark and Percy (1970–1), by David Hockney. Acrylic on canvas, 84 x 120 in. © David Hockney. Reproduced with permission of the copyright holder © Tate, London 2012.
- A Couple (1925), by Per Krohg, 65 x 81 cm. Ownership by Lillehammer Art Museum (Photo: Jacques Lathion). © DACS 2012. © Lillehammer Kunstmuseum/Jørn Hagen Artphoto.
- Branded (1992), by Jenny Saville. Reproduced with permission of the copyright holder. © 2001 Christie's Images Ltd. © Jenny Saville. Courtesy Gagosian Gallery.
- Romance (1921), by Cecile Walton. © The Scottish National Portrait Gallery.
- Self Portrait with Cigarette (1895), by Edvard Munch. National Gallery, Norway. © 2004 Munch Museum/Munch–Ellingsen Group, BONO, Oslo/DACS, London 2012.
- Last Sickness (1953), by Alice Neel. Oil on canvas, 30 x 22 in./76.2 x 55.9 cm. © Estate of Alice Neel. Courtesy of Robert Miller Gallery, New York. The Philadelphia Museum of Art holds the original; gift of Hartley S Neel and Richard Neel.

CHAPTER 7

- Branch Hill Pond, Hampstead Heath (1821–2), by John Constable. Oil on canvas. © Victoria and Albert Museum, London. Courtesy of the Trustees of the V&A.
- National Trust Handbook (2004), by permission.
- Resurrection (1996–9), by Anthony Green. © Anthony Green. Reproduced with permission of the copyright holder.
- Victorian terrace and parkland, Harewood House. Reproduced with permission of Harewood House Trust, Leeds.
- Reclining Figure, Arch Leg (1969–70) (bronze), by Henry Moore. Yorkshire Sculpture Park. © Henry Moore Foundation.
- Peine del Viento XVII (1990) (steel), by Eduardo Chillida. Yorkshire Sculpture Park. © Museo Chillida-Leku.
- Signs of the Times (1992) © Martin Parr/Magnum Photos. By permission of Magnum Photos.

CHAPTER 9

- Shadowlands (1992), by W Nicholson. Samuel French, London.
- Macbeth, by William Shakespeare, Muir K (ed.) (1962). The Arden Edition, Methuen, London.

- Catherine Hayes' Skirmishes. Reproduced by permission of Catherine Hayes. © Catherine Hayes. First published by Faber & Faber Ltd.
- James Robson's Mr Wonderful. Reproduced by permission of James Robson. © James Robson. First published by Samuel French Ltd.

INDEX

CPD with Radcliffe

You can now use a selection of our books to achieve CPD (Continuing Professional Development) points through directed reading.

We provide a free online form and downloadable certificate for your appraisal portfolio. Look for the CPD logo and register with us at: **www.radcliffehealth.com/cpd**

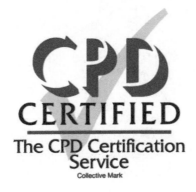

CPD with Radcliffe

You can now use a selection of our books to achieve CPD (Continuing Professional Development) points through directed reading.

We provide a free online form and downloadable certificate for your appraisal portfolio. Look for the CPD logo and register with us at www.radcliffehealth.com/cpd

The CPD Certification Service

9781846195655

9781846195655